IARC MONOGRAPHS
ON THE
EVALUATION OF THE CARCINOGENIC
RISK OF CHEMICALS TO MAN:

Some organochlorine pesticides

Volume 5

This publication represents the views of the
IARC Working Group on the
Evaluation of the Carcinogenic Risk of Chemicals to Man
which met in Lyon, 22-29 October 1973

IARC WORKING GROUP ON THE EVALUATION OF THE CARCINOGENIC RISK OF CHEMICALS
TO MAN: ORGANOCHLORINE PESTICIDES

Lyon, 22-29 October 1973

Members[1]

Dr D.C. Abbott, Senior Superintendant Environmental Chemistry, Laboratory
  of the Government Chemist, Department of Trade and Industry, Cornwall
  House, Stamford Street, London SE1 9NQ, UK

Dr R.D. Kimbrough[2], US Environmental Protection Agency, 4770 Buford Highway,
  Chamblee, Georgia 30341, USA

Dr R. Kroes, Head of the Department of Oncology, Laboratory for Pathology,
  Rijks Instituut voor de Volksgezondheid, Postbus 1, Bilthoven,
  The Netherlands

Professor M. Kuratsune, Department of Epidemiology, Medical School of Fukuoka,
  Kyushu University, Fukuoka, Japan

Dr J.L. Radomski, Professor of Pharmacology, University of Miami, School of
  Medicine, Box 875 Biscayne Annex, Miami, Florida 33152, USA

Dr U. Saffiotti, Associate Director for Carcinogenesis, Division of Cancer
  Cause and Prevention, National Cancer Institute, National Institutes
  of Health, Bethesda, Maryland 20014, USA (Chairman)

Dr M. Sharratt, Senior Medical Officer, Department of Health and Social
  Security, Alexander Fleming House, Elephant and Castle, London SE1 6BY,
  UK

Dr P. Shubik, Director, The Eppley Institute for Research in Cancer,
  University of Nebraska Medical Center, 42nd and Dewey Avenue, Omaha,
  Nebraska 68105, USA

Dr B. Terracini, Istituto di Anatomia e Istologia Patologica dell' Università
  di Torino, via Santena 7, Turin 10126, Italy (Vice Chairman)

---

[1]Unable to attend: Dr E.M. Poszarisski, Research Institute of Oncology,
68 Leningradskaya Street, Posjelok Pesochny 2, Leningrad, USSR; Dr E. Poulsen,
Director, Institute of Toxicology, Mørkhøjgaard, 19 Mørkhøj Bygade, DK-2860
Søborg, Denmark

[2]Present address: Centre for Disease Control, 9600 Clifton Road,
Atlanta, Georgia 30333, USA

Invited Guests

Dr L. Axelrod, US Environmental Protection Agency, Room 519, Waterside Mall, West Tower, 401 M Street SW, Washington DC 20460, USA

Miss I.B. Bertram, Deutsches Krebsforschungszentrum Institut für Toxikologie und Chemotherapie, Kirschnerstrasse 6, Postfach 449, D 6900 Heidelberg 1, Federal Republic of Germany

Mr J.C. Kolojeski, Attorney, US Environmental Protection Agency, Room 519, Waterside Mall, West Tower, 401 M Street SW, Washington DC 20460, USA

Dr K.E. McCaleb, Manager, Environmental Studies, Chemical Information Services, Stanford Research Institute, Menlo Park, California 94025, USA

Representative from the National Cancer Institute

Dr S. Siegel, Research Biologist, Carcinogen Bioassay and Programme Resource Branch, Carcinogenesis DCCP, National Cancer Institute, Landow Building, Room C 325, Bethesda, Maryland 20014, USA

Secretariat

Dr C. Agthe, Unit of Chemical Carcinogenesis (Secretary)

Dr H. Bartsch, Unit of Chemical Carcinogenesis

Dr N. Breslow, Unit of Epidemiology and Biostatistics

Dr A.J. Cohen, Consultant

Dr J. Copplestone, Vector Control and Biology Unit, WHO

Dr H.L. Falk, Consultant

Dr N. Napalkov, Chief, Cancer Unit, WHO

Mrs C. Partensky, Unit of Chemical Carcinogenesis

Mrs I. Peterschmitt, Unit of Chemical Carcinogenesis

Dr L. Tomatis, Chief, Unit of Chemical Carcinogenesis

Dr A.J. Tuyns, Unit of Epidemiology and Biostatistics

Mr E.A. Walker, Unit of Environmental Carcinogens

Mr J.D. Wilbourn, Unit of Chemical Carcinogenesis

CONTENTS

	Page
BACKGROUND AND PURPOSE OF THE IARC PROGRAMME ON THE EVALUATION OF THE CARCINOGENIC RISK OF CHEMICALS TO MAN	7
SCOPE OF THE MONOGRAPHS	7
MECHANISM FOR PRODUCING THE MONOGRAPHS	8
Priority for the preparation of monographs	8
Data on which the evaluation was based	9
The Working Group	9
GENERAL REMARKS ON THE EVALUATION	9
Purity of the compounds tested	9
Terminology	9
Response to **carcinogens**	10
Qualitative aspects	10
Dose-response relationships	10
Animal data in relation to the evaluation of risk to man	11
Evidence of human carcinogenicity	11
EXPLANATORY NOTES ON THE MONOGRAPHS	12
GENERAL REMARKS ON THE SUBSTANCES CONSIDERED IN THIS VOLUME	15
THE MONOGRAPHS	
Aldrin	25
Aramite^R	39
BHC (Technical grades) and lindane	47
Chlorobenzilate	75
DDT and associated substances	83
Dieldrin	125
Endrin	157
Heptachlor	173
Methoxychlor	193
Mirex	203

  Page

    Quintozene (Pentachloronitrobenzene) 211
    Terpene polychlorinates (Strobane^R) 219

APPENDIX 224

CUMULATIVE INDEX TO MONOGRAPHS 237

BACKGROUND AND PURPOSE OF THE IARC PROGRAMME ON THE EVALUATION OF THE CARCINOGENIC RISK OF CHEMICALS TO MAN

The International Agency for Research on Cancer (IARC) has initiated a programme for the evaluation of the carcinogenic risk of chemicals to man. This programme was supported by a Resolution of the Governing Council at its Ninth Session concerning the role of IARC in providing government authorities with expert, independent scientific opinion on environmental carcinogenesis. As one means to this end, the Governing Council recommended that IARC should continue to prepare monographs on the carcinogenic risk of individual chemicals to man.

In view of the importance of this programme and in order to expedite the production of monographs, the National Cancer Institute of the United States has provided IARC with additional funds for this purpose.

The aim of this programme is to arrive at and publish an objective evaluation of the available data through the deliberations of an international group of experts in chemical carcinogenesis, and to put into perspective the present state of knowledge with the final aim of evaluating the data in terms of possible human risk, as well as to indicate the need for research efforts to close the gaps in our knowledge.

SCOPE OF THE MONOGRAPHS

The monographs summarize the evidence for the carcinogenicity of individual chemicals. The data are compiled, reviewed and evaluated by a Working Group of experts. No recommendations are given concerning preventive measures or legislation, since these matters depend on risk-benefit evaluation, which seems best made by individual governments and/or international agencies such as WHO and ILO.

The first volume[1] covers a number of substances not belonging to a particular chemical group; the second volume[2] contains monographs on some inorganic and organometallic compounds; the third volume[3] covers a number of polycyclic aromatic hydrocarbons and heterocyclic compounds; and the fourth volume[4] is devoted to some miscellaneous alkylating agents. The present volume is devoted to some organochlorine pesticides.

As new data on chemicals for which monographs have already been written and new principles for evaluation become available, re-evaluations will be made at future meetings and revised monographs will be published as necessary. The monographs are being distributed to international and governmental agencies and will be available to industries and scientists dealing with these chemicals. They also form the basis of advice from IARC on carcinogenesis from these substances.

MECHANISM FOR PRODUCING THE MONOGRAPHS

As a first step, a list of chemicals for possible consideration by the Working Group is established. IARC then collects pertinent references regarding physico-chemical characteristics, production and use*, occurrence and analysis, and biological data** on these compounds. The material is summarized by an expert consultant or an IARC staff member, who prepares the first draft monograph, which in some cases is sent to another expert for comments. The drafts are circulated to all members of the Working Group about one month before the meeting, during which further additions to and deletions from the data are agreed upon and a final version of comments and evaluation on each compound is adopted.

Priority for the Preparation of Monographs

Priority is given mainly to chemicals belonging to groups for which some experimental evidence of carcinogenicity exists and for which there is evidence of human exposure. However, neither human exposure nor potential carcinogenicity can be judged until all the relevant data have been collected and examined in detail; and the inclusion of a particular compound in a monograph does not necessarily mean that the substance is considered to be carcinogenic. Equally, the fact that a substance has not yet been considered does not imply that it is without carcinogenic hazard.

---

* Data provided by Chemical Information Services, Stanford Research Institute, Menlo Park, California, USA

** In the collection of original data reference was made to CBAC profile sheets and to the publications "Survey of compounds which have been tested for carcinogenic activity" [5,6,7,8,9,10,11].

Data on which the Evaluation is Based

With regard to the biological data, only published articles and papers already accepted for publication are reviewed. Every effort is made to cover the whole literature, but some studies may have been inadvertently overlooked. The monographs are not intended to be a full review of the literature, and they contain only data considered relevant to the Committee. Research workers who are aware of important data (published or accepted for publication) which may influence the evaluation are invited to make them available to the Unit of Chemical Carcinogenesis of the International Agency for Research on Cancer, Lyon, France.

The Working Group

The members of the Working Group who participated in the consideration of particular substances are listed at the beginning of each publication. The members of the Working Group serve in their individual capacities as scientists, and not as representatives of their governments or of any organization with which they are affiliated.

GENERAL REMARKS ON THE EVALUATION

Purity of the Compounds Tested

In any evaluation of biological data with respect to a possible carcinogenic risk, particular attention must be paid to the purity of the chemicals tested and to their stability under conditions of storage or administration. Information on purity and stability is given, when available, in the Monographs.

Terminology

The term "chemical carcinogenesis" in its widely accepted sense is used to indicate the induction or enhancement of neoplasia by chemicals. It is recognized that, in the strict etymological sense, this term means the induction of cancer. However, common usage has led to its employment to denote the induction of various types of neoplasms. The terms "tumourigen", "oncogen" and "blastomogen" have all been used synonymously with "carcinogen", although occasionally "tumourigen" has been used specifically to denote the induction of benign tumours.

Response to Carcinogens

For present purposes, in general, no distinction is made between the induction of tumours and the enhancement of tumour incidence, although it is noted that there may be fundamental differences in mechanisms that will eventually be elucidated.

The response in experimental animals to a carcinogen may take several forms:

(a) a significant increase in the incidence of one or more of the same types of neoplasms as found in control animals;

(b) the occurrence of types of neoplasms not observed in control animals;

(c) a decreased latent period as compared with control animals.

Qualitative Aspects

The qualitative nature of neoplasia has been much discussed. In many instances both benign and malignant tumours are induced by chemical carcinogens. There are so far few recorded instances in which only benign tumours are induced by chemicals that have been studied extensively. Their occurrence in experimental systems has been taken to indicate the possibility of an increased risk of malignant tumours also.

In experimental carcinogenesis, the type of cancer seen can be the same as that recorded in human studies (e.g., bladder cancer in man, monkeys, dogs and hamsters after administration of 2-naphthylamine). In other instances, however, a chemical can induce other types of neoplasms or neoplasms at different sites in various species (e.g., benzidine, which induces hepatic carcinoma in the rat, but bladder carcinoma in man).

Dose-Response Relationships

Dose-response studies are important in the evaluation of human and animal carcinogenesis. The confidence with which a carcinogenic effect can be established is strengthened by the observation of an increasing incidence of neoplasms with increasing exposure.

Animal Data in Relation to the Evaluation of Risk to Man

At the present time no attempt can be made to interpret the animal data directly in terms of human risk since no objective criteria are available to do so. The critical assessment of the validity of the animal data given in these Monographs is intended to assist national and/or international authorities to make decisions concerning preventive measures or legislation. In this connection, attention is drawn to WHO recommendations in relation to food additives[12], drugs[13] and occupational **carcinogens**[14].

Evidence of Human Carcinogenicity

Evaluation of the carcinogenic risk to man of suspected environmental agents rests on purely observational studies. Such studies require sufficient variation in the levels of human exposure to allow a meaningful relationship between cancer incidence and exposure to a given chemical to be established. Difficulties in isolating the effects of individual agents arise, however, since populations are exposed to multiple carcinogens.

The initial suggestion of a relationship between an agent and disease often comes from case reports of patients who have had similar exposures. Variations and time trends in regional or national cancer incidence, or their correlation with regional or national 'exposure' levels, may also provide valuable insights. Such observations by themselves, however, cannot in most circumstances be regarded as conclusive evidence of carcinogenicity. The most satisfactory epidemiological method is to compare the cancer risk (adjusted for age, sex and other confounding variables) among groups or cohorts, or among individuals exposed to various levels of the agent in question with that among control groups not so exposed. Ideally this is accomplished directly, by following such groups forward in time (prospectively) to determine time relationships, dose-response relationships and other aspects of cancer induction. Large cohorts and long observation periods are required to provide sufficient cases for a statistically valid comparison.

An alternative to prospective investigation is to assemble cohorts from past records and to evaluate their subsequent morbidity or mortality by means of medical histories and death certificates. Such occupational carcinogens as nickel, β-naphthylamine, asbestos and benzidine have been confirmed by this method. Another method is to compare the past exposures of a defined group of cancer cases with those of control samples from the hospital or general population. This does not provide an absolute measure of carcinogenic risk but can indicate the relative risks associated with different levels of exposure. The indirect means (e.g., interviews or tissue residues) used to measure exposures which may have commenced many years before can constitute a major source of error. Nevertheless such "case/control" studies can often isolate one factor from several suspected agents. The carcinogenic effect of this substance could then be confirmed by cohort studies.

EXPLANATORY NOTES ON THE MONOGRAPHS

In sections 1, 2 and 3 of each monograph, except for minor remarks, the data are recorded as given by the author, whereas the comments by the Working Group are given in section 4, headed "Comments on Data Reported and Evaluation".

Chemical and Physical Data (section 1)

The most important chemical synonyms and trade names are recorded in this section.

Chemical and physical properties include data that might be relevant to carcinogenicity (for example, lipid solubility) and those that concern identification. Where applicable, data on solubility, volatility and stability are indicated. All data in this section, except those for "Technical products and impurities", refer to the pure substances.

Production, Use, Occurrence and Analysis (section 2)

With regard to the data on use and occurrence of chemicals presented in the monographs, IARC has collaborated with the Stanford Research Institute, USA, with the support of the National Cancer Institute of the United States, in order to obtain production figures of chemicals and their patterns of use. These data more commonly refer to the United States and Western Europe than to other countries, solely as a result of the availability to the

Working Group of more data from these countries than from others. It should not be implied that these nations are the sole sources or even the major sources of any individual chemical.

In some countries, there are also legal restrictions on the conditions under which certain carcinogens, suspect chemicals and pesticides can be handled. Examples of these are given in section 2.2 when such information was available to the Working Group.

It is hoped that in future revisions of these Monographs, more information on use and legislation can be made available to IARC from other countries.

Biological Data Relevant to the Evaluation of Carcinogenic Risk to Man (section 3)

As pointed out earlier in this introduction, the monographs are not intended to consider all studies reported in the literature. Although every effort was made to review the whole literature, some studies were purposely omitted (a) because of their inadequacy, as judged from previously described criteria[15,16,17,18] (e.g., too short a duration, too few animals, poor survival or too small a dose); (b) because they only confirmed findings which have already been fully described; or (c) because they were judged irrelevant for the purpose of the evaluation. However, in certain cases, reference is made to studies which did not meet established criteria of adequacy, particularly when this information was considered a useful supplement to other reports or when it may have been the only data available. This does not, however, imply acceptance of the adequacy of experimental designs in these cases.

In general, the data recorded in this section are summarized as given by the author; however, certain shortcomings of reporting or of experimental design are also mentioned, and minor comments by the Working Group are given in parentheses.

The essential critical comments by the Working Group are made in section 4 ("Comments on Data Reported and Evaluation").

Carcinogenicity and related studies in animals (3.1)

Mention is usually made of all routes of administration by which the compound has been tested and of all species in which relevant tests have been carried out. In some cases where similar results were obtained by several authors, reference is made to a summary article. Quantitative data are given in so far as they will enable the reader to realize the order of magnitude of the effective doses. In general the doses are indicated as they appear in the original paper; sometimes conversions have been made for better comparison, and these are given in parentheses.

Other relevant biological data (3.2)

The reporting of metabolic data is restricted to studies showing the metabolic fate of the chemical in animals and man. Comparison of animal and human data is made when possible. Other metabolic information (e.g., absorption, storage and excretion) is given when the Working Group considered that it would enable the reader to have a better understanding of the fate of the compound in the body. When the carcinogenicity of known metabolites has been tested, this also is reported.

Data on toxicity are included occasionally, if considered relevant.

Observations in man (3.3)

Epidemiological studies are summarized. Clinical and other observations in man have been reviewed, when relevant.

Comments on Data Reported and Evaluation (section 4)

This section gives the critical view of the Working Group on the data reported. It should be read in conjunction with the data recorded.

Animal data (4.1)

In general, the animal species and routes of administration mentioned here are those in which the carcinogenicity of the substances was adequately investigated. In the case of inadequate studies, when mentioned, comments to that effect are included. Tumour sites are usually mentioned.

Human data (4.2)

The significance of epidemiological studies and case reports is evaluated.

GENERAL REMARKS ON THE SUBSTANCES CONSIDERED IN THIS VOLUME

This volume of monographs is devoted to twelve organochlorine pesticides. The compounds considered were selected on the criteria of the availability of experimental studies suggesting carcinogenicity. The fact that a substance has been considered does not necessarily mean that it is carcinogenic, nor that a related substance which has not been considered in the present volume is necessarily non-carcinogenic.

The extensive environmental distribution of organochlorine pesticides has been well documented, and several reviews are available[19,20,21,22].

Many of these organochlorine compounds are highly stable and persist in the environment. Rates of biochemical transformation vary for different compounds and different environmental circumstances, and the time required for a 50% change in concentration may range from weeks to years; the period may be longer still in abiotic components of the environment. Gamma-BHC is more easily transformed into less toxic substances than is the beta-isomer, which is more stable. The primary metabolic products of aldrin and heptachlor, dieldrin and heptachlor epoxide, respectively, are very stable substances, as is DDE, a metabolic product of DDT.

Organochlorine compounds are generally only very slightly soluble in water; on the other hand, they are very soluble in lipids. For this reason they tend to be stored in animal tissues at levels that depend on the intake and the metabolic peculiarities of the species concerned. Some aquatic organisms may acquire levels of organochlorine compounds exceeding 10 000 times that in the water in which they live[20]. An additional property associated with their low solubility in water is a tendency to adsorb onto suspended particulate matter in water, on bottom sediments and on organic matter in soil.

Most organochlorine insecticides have a low vapour pressure, but when an extensive surface is exposed, appreciable amounts of vapour can find their way into the air by volatilization or co-distillation with water. Direct aerial application or spray-drift can also contribute to carriage by air. These vapours in turn condense on colloidal particles suspended in air or coalesce into aerosol droplets and thus can be transported over considerable distances. This may be one of the most important mechanisms by which DDT and also some other pollutants are transported from the land to the sea[23].

While, for the majority of the general population, the body content of organochlorine pesticides is probably derived mainly from the diet[24,25], other sources in the immediate environment, such as occupational exposures, domestic uses, thermal vaporizers or public health uses, may provide an important contribution for some smaller populations or for individuals. This is particularly true in the cases of DDT and BHC. The contributions from drinking-water or from ambient air to the intake of these compounds by the general population are of minor importance.

Methods of organochlorine pesticide residue analysis

In general, an analytical method which is adequate for the determination of a pesticide residue on a commodity to which the pesticide has been applied in a supervised trial is not necessarily satisfactory for determination of the same pesticide when samples of unknown treatment history are being examined. Similarly, a procedure that is suitable for assessing whether a specified food commodity complies with a recommended tolerance for a particular pesticide may not be applicable to other commodities, nor to other pesticides on the original commodity.

In addition, variations in available apparatus, reagents and experimental conditions, the presence of other pesticides or their metabolites or the presence of other interfering compounds of either natural or synthetic origin make it impossible to specify any one procedure that will always satisfactorily determine the residue of a particular pesticide in any substrate. Thus, it is usually necessary to adapt a generally acceptable procedure to suit the particular circumstances involved (e.g., the reason for the analysis, the nature of the sample, the nature of the residue and the type and extent of interference likely to be met). In addition, some form of positive identification of the residue is desirable.

Several satisfactory gas-chromatographic multi-residue methods are available for the detection and determination of residues of organochlorine pesticides. Extraction from the sample with a suitable solvent (e.g., hexane, acetone-hexane, propan-2-ol, benzene, acetonitrile, dimethylformamide, etc.,) is generally followed by clean-up stages for the removal of coextracted fatty or other interfering material. These stages employ solvent partition procedures and/or columnar adsorbent treatment. The residues remaining in the purified extract are then detected and determined by gas-liquid chromatography (GLC) on at least two stationary phases of differing polarity, by electron-capture or by micro-coulometric detection systems. Thin-layer or paper chromatography and/or chemical conversion reactions followed by further GLC examination are often used, when required, to confirm the identity of the observed residues.

Some references to analytical procedures are given in the appropriate sections, but for general purposes the Pesticide Analytical Manual[26] provides a valuable starting point, according to IUPAC[27]. Clean-up procedures are detailed by Faubert Maunder et al.[28], Wood[29] and Mills et al.[30]. Abbott et al.[25,31] have described the procedures used for examining total diet and human fat samples; this paper also gives details of techniques used to confirm the identity of the residues.

Methods of pesticide residue analysis have been reviewed recently[32].

Experimental data

The amount of available information concerning the effects of organochlorine pesticides in laboratory animals varied greatly between compounds. The Working Group was aware that there is unpublished information and work in progress on long-term studies on the materials considered in this volume, but this could not be taken into consideration (see preamble, p. 9). Adequacy of reporting also varied within a wide range. In some cases reproducibility of results could be evaluated, while in others only small-scale studies giving evidence of carcinogenicity had been carried out. Although exposure to organochlorine pesticides can be induced by the respiratory route, it was particularly noted that no long-term studies using this route have been reported. When available, the composition of the tested material is given.

For several organochlorine compounds evidence of carcinogenicity is based mainly on the production of parenchymal liver-cell tumours in mice.

The Working Group noted that there is considerable variation in the interpretation of the histological and biological characteristics of these tumours. In some instances, authors have not given sufficient details to allow an evaluation of the degree of malignancy of these tumours, and, in addition, the use of the term "hepatoma" has created confusion, as it covers tumours which have been described both as benign and/or malignant. As a rule the terminology and histological description of the tumours, as given by the authors, are reported in the Monographs.

Other biological effects

For several of the organochlorine pesticides considered in the present volume, other biological effects have been demonstrated; these compounds may persist in the environment and in tissues of animals and man, cross the placental barrier, induce microsomal enzymes and produce neurotoxic effects.

Enzyme induction occurs mostly in the liver but has also been studied in lung, intestine and other organ systems, where it occurs to a lesser extent. Enzyme induction has been found in all mammalian species studied. The extent of induction varies considerably with age, sex, species and genetic constitution. This subject has been reviewed[33,34,35]

Such increased enzyme activity declines within a few weeks following the disappearance of the inducer from the organism. However, organochlorine pesticides which are persistent in the organism may lead to a more prolonged induction of enzyme systems. Their persistence in the environment may further contribute to the maintenance of the induced stage. Enzyme induction results in an increased metabolism not only of exogenous compounds but also of endogenous compounds, e.g., steroids. The increase in enzyme activity leads to a greater rate of production of metabolites, and these may be either more or less toxic/carcinogenic than the parent compound.

Epidemiological data

In contrast with the large amount of information available from experiments on animals, there is remarkably little data on humans. This is undoubtedly due in part to the difficulties inherent in epidemiological investigations on environmental chemicals (see p. 11).

It was regretted that no adequate systematic correlation studies have been made since the introduction of these materials into the environment, to determine whether meaningful associations can be demonstrated between exposure levels and changes in cancer incidences.

Epidemiological studies utilizing occupational exposure have been carried out for only a few pesticides.

References

1. IARC (1972) *IARC Monographs on the Evaluation of Carcinogenic Risk of Chemicals to Man*, 1, Lyon

2. IARC (1973) *IARC Monographs on the Evaluation of Carcinogenic Risk of Chemicals to Man, 2, Some Inorganic and Organometallic Compounds*, Lyon

3. IARC (1973) *IARC Monographs on the Evaluation of Carcinogenic Risk of Chemicals to Man, 3, Certain Polycyclic Aromatic Hydrocarbons and Heterocyclic Compounds*, Lyon

4. IARC (1974) *IARC Monographs on the Evaluation of Carcinogenic Risk of Chemicals to Man, 4, Some Aromatic Amines, Hydrazine and Related Substances, N-nitroso Compounds and Miscellaneous Alkylating Agents*, Lyon

5. Hartwell, J.L. (1951) *Survey of compounds which have been tested for carcinogenic activity*, Washington, DC, US Government Printing Office (Public Health Service Publication No. 149)

6. Shubik, P. & Hartwell, J.L. (1957) *Survey of compounds which have been tested for carcinogenic activity*, Washington, DC, US Government Printing Office (Public Health Service Publication No. 149: Supplement 1)

7. Shubik, P. & Hartwell, J.L. (1969) *Survey of compounds which have been tested for carcinogenic activity*, Washington, DC, US Government Printing Office (Public Health Service Publication No. 149: Supplement 2)

8. Carcinogenesis Program National Cancer Institute (1973) *Survey of compounds which have been tested for carcinogenic activity*, Washington, DC, US Government Printing Office (Public Health Service Publication No. 149: 1961-1967)

9. Thompson, J.I. & Co. (1971) *Survey of compounds which have been tested for carcinogenic activity*, Washington, DC, US Government Printing Office (Public Health Service Publication No. 149: 1968-1969)

10. Carcinogenesis Program National Cancer Institute (1974) *Survey of compounds which have been tested for carcinogenic activity*, Washington, DC, US Government Printing Office (Public Health Service Publication No. 149: 1970-1971) (in press)

11. Carcinogenesis Program National Cancer Institute ( ) *Survey of compounds which have been tested for carcinogenic activity*, Washington, DC, US Government Printing Office (Public Health Service Publication No. 149: 1972-1973) (in preparation)

12. WHO (1961) Fifth Report of the Joint FAO/WHO Expert Committee on Food Additives. Evaluation of carcinogenic hazard of food additives. Wld Hlth Org. techn. Rep. Ser., No. 220, pp. 5, 18, 19

13. WHO (1969) Report of a WHO Scientific Group. Principles for the testing and evaluation of drugs for carcinogenicity. Wld Hlth Org. techn. Rep. Ser., No. 426, pp. 19, 21, 22

14. WHO (1964) Report of a WHO Expert Committee. Prevention of Cancer. Wld Hlth Org. techn. Rep. Ser., No. 276, pp. 29, 30

15. WHO (1958) Second Report of the Joint FAO/WHO Expert Committee on Food Additives. Procedures for the testing of intentional food additives to establish their safety for use. Wld Hlth Org. techn. Rep. Ser., No. 144

16. WHO (1961) Fifth Report of the Joint FAO/WHO Expert Committee on Food Additives. Evaluation of carcinogenic hazard of food additives. Wld Hlth Org. techn. Rep. Ser., No. 220

17. WHO (1967) Scientific Group. Procedures for investigating intentional and unintentional food additives. Wld Hlth Org. techn. Rep. Ser., No. 348

18. UICC (1969) Carcinogenicity testing. UICC techn. Rep. Ser., Vol. 2

19. US Department of Health, Education and Welfare (1969) Report of the Secretary's Commission on Pesticides and their Relationship to Environmental Health, Parts I & II, Washington, DC, US Government Printing Office

20. Agricultural Research Council (1970) Third Report of the Research Committee on Toxic Chemicals, London, HMSO

21. Gillet, J.W., ed. (1970) The biological impact of pesticides in the environment. In: Proceedings of a Symposium, Oregon State University, Cornwallis, Oregon, 1970, Cornwallis, Oregon, Oregon State University Press

22. Kaloyanova-Simeonova, F. & Fournier, E. (1971) Les Pesticides et l'Homme, Paris, Masson

23. IMCO/FAO/UNESCO/WHO/WMO/IAEA/UN Joint Group of Experts on the Scientific Aspects of Marine Pollution (GESAMP) (1971) Report of the Third Session, Rome, 1970, Geneva, WHO (unpublished document WHO/W. POLL/71.8; GESAMP III/19) (to be published)

24. Campbell, J.E., Richardson, L.A. & Schafer, M.L. (1965) Insecticide residues in the human diet. Arch. environm. Hlth, 10, 831

25. Abbott, D.C., Collins, G.B. & Goulding, R. (1972) Organochlorine pesticide residues in human fat in the United Kingdom 1969-71. Brit. med. J., ii, 553

26. Barry, H.C., Hindley, J.G. & Johnson, L.Y. (1963-1972) Pesticide Analytical Manual, Vols 1 & 2, Washington DC, US Government Printing Office (Food & Drug Administration, US Department of Health, Education & Welfare) (revised periodically)

27. IUPAC (1970) Report of the Fourth Meeting of the Commission on Pesticide Residue Analysis. J. Ass. off. analyt. Chem., 53, 1004

28. Faubert Maunder, M.J., de, Egan, H., Godly, E.W., Hammond, E.W., Roburn, J. & Thomson, J. (1964) Clean-up of animal fats and dairy products for the analysis of chlorinated pesticide residues. Analyst, 89, 168

29. Wood, N.F. (1969) Extraction and clean-up of organochlorine pesticide residues by column chromatography. Analyst, 94, 399

30. Mills, P.A., Bong, B.A., Kamps, L.R. & Burke, J.A. (1972) Elution solvent system for Florisil column clean-up in organochlorine pesticide residue analysis. J. Ass. off. analyt. Chem., 55, 39

31. Abbott, D.C., Holmes, D.C. & Tatton, J.O'G. (1969) Pesticide residues in the total diet in England and Wales 1966-67. II. Organo-chlorine pesticide residues in the total diet. J. Sci. Fd Agric., 20, 245

32. Ruzicka, J.H.A. & Abbott, D.t. (1973) Pesticide residue analysis. Talanta, 20 (in press)

33. Conney, A.H. (1965) Enzyme induction and drug toxicity. In: Brodie, B.B. & Gillette, J.R., eds, Drugs and Enzymes, Oxford, London, Pergamon, p. 277

34. Gelboin, H.V. (1967) Carcinogens, enzyme induction and gene action. Adv. Cancer Res., 10, 1

35. Gillette, J.R., Conney, A.H., Cosmides, G.J., Estabrook, R.W., Fonts, J.R. & Mannering, G.J. (1969) Microsomes and Drug Oxidations, New York, Academic Press, pp. 1-547

SOME ORGANOCHLORINE PESTICIDES

ALDRIN

Aldrin is the common name approved by the International Standards Organization (except in Canada, Denmark and USSR) for the product containing not less than 95% of 1,2,3,4,10,10-hexachloro-1,4,4a,8,8a-hexahydro-<u>exo</u>-1,4-<u>endo</u>-5,8-dimethanonaphthalene. In Canada, aldrin refers to the pure compound (which is known as HHDN in Great Britain). Two reviews on this compound are available (FAO/WHO, 1967, 1968).

1. Chemical and Physical Data

1.1 <u>Synonyms and trade names</u>

Chem. Abstr. No.: 309-00-2

Compound 118; ENT 15,949; 1,2,3,4,10,10-hexachloro-1,4,4a,8,8a-hexahydro-<u>endo</u>,<u>exo</u>-1,4:5,8-dimethanonaphthalene; hexachlorohexahydro-<u>endo-exo</u>-dimethanonaphthalene; 1,2,3,4,10,10-hexachloro-1,4,4a,5,8,8a-hexahydro-<u>endo</u>-1,4,-<u>exo</u>-5,8-dimethanonaphthalene; 1,2,3,4,10,10-hexachloro-1,4,4a,5,8,8a-hexahydro-1,4-<u>endo-exo</u>-5,8-dimethanonaphthalene; 1,2,3,4,10,10-hexachloro-1,4,4a,5,8,8a-hexahydro-<u>exo</u>-1,4-<u>endo</u>-5,8-dimethanonaphthalene; HHDN

1.2 <u>Chemical formula and molecular weight</u>

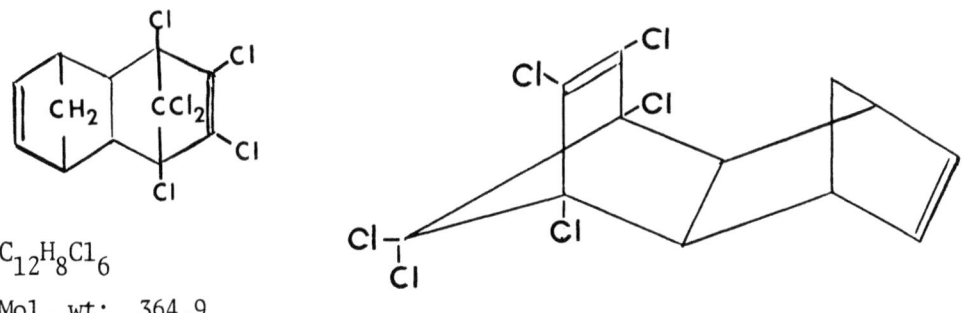

$C_{12}H_8Cl_6$
Mol. wt: 364.9

1.3. <u>Chemical and physical properties of the pure substance</u>

(a) <u>Description</u>: White, crystalline, odourless solid

(b) <u>Melting-point</u>: 104-104.5°C

(c) <u>Solubility</u>: Very soluble in most organic solvents; practically insoluble in water (0.027 mg/l)

(d) <u>Volatility</u>: Vapour pressure is 2.31 x 10^{-5} mm Hg at 20°C

(e) <u>Chemical reactivity</u>: Stable to heat and in the presence of inorganic and organic bases; stable to the action of hydrated metal chlorides and mild acids. Epoxidation of aldrin with peracetic or perbenzoic acid forms the 6,7-epoxy derivative, dieldrin; under most environmental conditions aldrin is gradually converted to dieldrin. The unchlorinated ring is attacked by oxidizing agents and strong acids.

1.4 <u>Technical products and impurities</u>

The technical product is a tan to dark-brown solid, melting between 49 and 60°C. In 1967, the composition of technical aldrin was reported to be as follows: 90.5% hexachlorohexahydrodimethanonaphthalene (HHDN), 3.5% other polychlorohexahydrodimethanonaphthalene (isodrin), 0.5% hexachlorotetrahydromethanoindene (chlordane), 0.2% hexachlorocyclopentadiene (HCCPD), 0.6% hexachlorobutadiene, 0.5% octachlorocyclopentene, <0.1% hexachloroethane, 0.1% HHDN diadduct, <0.1% bicycloheptadiene (BCH), 0.3% toluene and 3.6% other compounds (primarily a complex mixture of compounds formed by polymerization of HCCPD and BCH during the aldrin reaction) (FAO/WHO, 1968).

Aldrin is available in the United States as a technical grade product containing 95% minimum active ingredient (equivalent to 90.3% of HHDN and 4.7% of other insecticidally-active, related compounds) (Frear, 1972; Whetstone, 1964). It is formulated into emulsifiable concentrates, wettable powders, dusts, granules and mixtures with fertilizers.

2. <u>Production, Use, Occurrence and Analysis</u>

2.1 <u>Production and use</u>[1]

Aldrin was first synthesized in the laboratory in about 1948 (Whetstone, 1964); commercial production in the US was first reported in

---

[1] Data from Chemical Information Services, Stanford Research Institute, USA

1950 (US Tariff Commission, 1951). Aldrin is made by the Diels-Alder reaction of hexachlorocyclopentadiene with bicycloheptadiene (Whetstone, 1964).

Only one company manufactures aldrin in the US, and it has been estimated that this manufacturer sold 4-5.4 million kg of aldrin in 1962 (Whetstone, 1964). Another source has estimated that 4.5 million kg of aldrin were produced in 1971 (Johnson, 1972).

Imports of aldrin through the principal US customs districts were reported to have been 96 thousand kg in 1967 (US Tariff Commission, 1968).

The following European countries were reported to be producing aldrin in 1972 or 1973 (the number of producing companies is given in parentheses): Belgium (1), Federal Republic of Germany (1), France (2), Italy (2), The Netherlands (1), United Kingdom (1) (Chemical Information Services Ltd., 1973; Ragno, 1972). In 1972, Japan was reported to have seven suppliers of aldrin and aldrin formulations, some of which may also be producers of aldrin (Chemical Daily Co., 1973). Imports into Japan were reported to have been 143 thousand kg in 1970 (Hayashi, 1971).

Annual world production of aldrin in 1967 amounted to 4,500 kg (FAO/WHO, 1968).

The only known use for aldrin is as an insecticide, and one significant outlet is in the treatment of soil around structures for the control of termites. In 1972, one source estimated that 80% of the combined US production of aldrin and dieldrin was used on corn crops and that about 10% was used for termite control (Anon., 1972). As of May 15, 1970 aldrin was approved in the US for use on 49 agricultural crops (including several kinds of seed) and for soil treatment around certain fruits, nuts and vegetables. Tolerances for residues of aldrin were set at 0-0.1 ppm on many of the raw agricultural products, and restrictions were placed on the use of treated seeds (US Environmental Protection Agency, 1970).

The approved uses for aldrin have been reviewed by the controlling US government agencies several times during the past few years because of the persistence of its degradation product, dieldrin, in the environment. The latest of these reviews was still in progress in October 1973.

Aldrin usage in California, a major agricultural state, was reported to have been nearly 22.7 thousand kg in 1971 - almost 90% of this was used for control of insects in structures (California Department of Agriculture, 1972) - and 14.5 thousand kg in 1972 when over 77% was used for the same purpose (California Department of Agriculture, 1973).

In July 1973, the US Environmental Protection Agency proposed a list of toxic pollutants, which includes aldrin (US Environmental Protection Agency, 1973). If this list is adopted, effluent standards restricting or prohibiting discharges of aldrin into streams may come into effect.

The quantities of this chemical used in, or sold for, agricultural purposes in 1970 were reported to be as follows (thousand kg): Burma (4.2); Canada (18.5); Colombia (198.5); El Salvador (21.9); Ghana (15.5); Iceland (0.1); Italy (2.765); Madagascar (3.5); Ryukyu Islands (9.1); and Uruguay (9.0) (FAO, 1972).

An indication of possible uses of aldrin can be derived from the FAO/WHO recommended residue limits for aldrin in the following food products: asparagus, broccoli, Brussels sprouts, cabbages, cauliflowers, cucumbers, aubergines, horseradishes, onions, parsnips, peppers, pimentoes, radishes, radish tops, fruits (including citrus), rice, potatoes, carrots, lettuces, milk and milk products, raw cereals and eggs (FAO/WHO, 1973).

The use of aldrin has been banned in Japan (Ogata, 1972), Norway (Stenersen, 1972) and the USSR (Melnikov & Shevchenko, 1971). The Federal Republic of Germany is allowing aldrin to be used in vineyards until the end of 1974 (BBLF, 1972), and it has limited uses in the United Kingdom (UK Ministry of Agriculture, Fisheries & Food, 1973). The sale of aldrin for agricultural purposes was recently prohibited in Italy.

2.2 Occurrence

(a) Air:

During an extensive monitoring of the ambient air, aldrin could be detected in only 1 of 875 samples taken in 9 localities of the US at a level of 8.0 ng/m^3 (Stanley et al., 1971). In a small number of samples taken in agricultural communities, concentrations ranged from 0.1-4 ng/m^3 (Tabor, 1966).

(b) <u>Soil and water</u>

Many studies of the aldrin residue levels in agricultural soils have been carried out (Gish, 1970; McCaskill et al., 1970; Saha & Sumner, 1971; Sand et al., 1972; Trautmann et al., 1968; Wiersma et al., 1972a,b). Aldrin was found less often and in smaller quantities than was dieldrin, due to epoxidation of aldrin to dieldrin in soil (Elgar, 1966; Lichtenstein et al., 1964, 1970). Average dieldrin concentrations ranged from 0.001-0.02 ppm (McCaskill et al., 1970; Wiersma et al., 1972b).

Decker et al. (1965) showed that application of up to 25 lb aldrin/acre of corn soils resulted in the retention of 10% of the applied level after 4 years, this remaining mainly in the form of dieldrin.

Aldrin has been detected in the water of Lake Utah (over 1 ppb) (Bradshaw et al., 1972) and in samples of river water taken near the factory of a primary manufacturer of endrin and heptachlor (Barthel et al., 1969). A maximum of 0.03 µg/l has been found in ocean surface slicks (Seba & Corcoran, 1969).

(c) <u>Food</u>

Aldrin is readily converted into dieldrin in plants and animals; as a consequence it is rarely found as such in food. In milk fat an average level of 0.001 ppm has been detected (Duggan, 1967), and in milk, butter and cheese, 0.027 ppm (Tolle et al., 1972).

In total-diet samples collected in the US aldrin was detected in trace amounts in dairy products, meat, fish and poultry, grains and cereals and fruits and vegetables (Corneliussen, 1969; Cummings, 1966; Duggan et al., 1966, 1967; Martin & Duggan, 1968). Less than 0.001 ppm have been found in meat, fish and poultry (Cummings, 1966) and 0.002 ppm in grains and cereals (Cummings, 1966); in fruits maximum values of 0.02 and 0.015 ppm (Duggan et al., 1966; Martin & Duggan, 1968) have been found.

In the US, Duggan & Lipscomb (1969) and Duggan & Corneliussen (1972) found that the average daily intake of aldrin from food ranged from 0.04-0.0001 µg/kg bw/day for the period 1965-1970. The 6-year average intake was 0.01 µg/kg bw/day.

No separate acceptable daily intake (ADI) was set for aldrin by the joint FAO/WHO Meeting on pesticide residues in food, although a total dieldrin and aldrin ADI of 0-0.0001 mg/kg bw/day has been recommended (FAO/WHO, 1971).

In the US a threshold limit value of 0.25 mg/m^3 has been established for an 8-hour time-weighted average occupational exposure (US Code of Federal Regulations, 1972).

2.3 Analysis

A general approach to the analysis of organochlorine pesticides has been given in the preamble (p. 16).

Identification by mass spectrometry has been described by Mumma & Kantner (1966), and gas chromatography has been used for analyses of animal feed by Begliomini & Fravolini (1971). A method for extraction from air is described by Aue & Teli (1971).

Further analytical methods can be found in the references cited in the section on "Occurrence".

3. Biological Data Relevant to the Evaluation of Carcinogenic Risk to Man

3.1 Carcinogenicity and related studies in animals

(a) Oral administration

Mouse: A group of 215 C3HeB/Fe mice divided approximately equally by sex were fed a diet containing 10 ppm aldrin for 2 years, after which all survivors were killed. A similar group of 217 untreated mice was used as a control. Average survival time was 51.8 weeks in treated mice compared with 59.8 in the controls. Liver tumours diagnosed as hepatic-cell adenomas and described as 'extending from very benign lesions to borderline carcinomas' were found in 38 treated and 9 control mice. On average, test mice developed hepatic tumours in 80 weeks and control mice in 89 weeks (Davis & Fitzhugh, 1962). (Evaluation of this study was not possible because of poor survival rate, lack of detailed pathology, loss of information due to inability to autopsy a large percentage of animals and failure to treat the results in males and females separately.)

Rat: Aldrin (95% pure) was fed to groups of 40 male and 40 female rats at concentrations of 0, 2.5, 12.5 and 25 ppm in the diet for 2 years. Only liver pathology was reported. The liver:body weight ratio was increased with the administration of levels of 2.5 ppm and above in males and of 12.5 ppm in females. No reference was made to the occurrence of tumours (Treon & Cleveland, 1955).

Groups of 12 male and 12 female Osborne-Mendel rats were fed diets containing 0, 0.5, 2, 10, 50, 100 or 150 ppm recrystallized aldrin for 2 years. Survival rates decreased at 50 ppm and above. Liver:body weight ratio was increased at all dose levels with obvious dose response at 50 ppm and above. Considering together the groups given 0.5, 2 or 10 ppm aldrin (i.e., the groups showing survival rates at 2 years comparable to those of the controls), the number of tumour-bearing animals was 25/60 in the treated animals compared with 3/17 in the controls. Among treated rats, 12 developed lymphomas (9 of which were located in the lungs), 13 had mammary tumours (malignant in 4 rats), 2 had fibrosarcomas and 3 had tumours at other sites. The 3 tumour-bearing control rats, had, respectively, a pulmonary lymphoma, a benign mammary tumour and a tumour at another site (Fitzhugh et al., 1964).

(Fitzhugh et al. considered their results to be evidence of 'some general type of effect that increased tumour production, without causing any single type of tumour to predominate'. However, the difference between 25/60 tumour-bearing rats given 0.5-10 ppm aldrin and 3/17 tumour-bearing controls is of doubtful significance (χ^2 = 2.34, P>0.05).)

Two groups of 30 male and 30 female Osborne-Mendel rats were fed a diet containing 5 ppm technical (95%) aldrin for 24-27 months. Forty-nine of the 60 treated rats were alive after 18 months compared with 48 of 60 controls. Mammary tumours (all benign, with one exception) were found in

11 treated and 12 control rats. Tumours at other sites in either sex were found in 4 treated and 3 control rats. No liver-cell tumours were found (Deichmann et al., 1967).

Groups of 50 male and 50 female Osborne-Mendel rats were fed diets containing 20, 30 or 50 ppm technical aldrin (95%) for lifespan and were compared to two control groups of 100 rats of each sex. Survival rate was not affected in males, while in females the mean survival time was 19.5 months in controls, 18.7 months in those receiving 20 ppm, 18.5 months with 30 ppm and 13.0 months with 50 ppm. The proportion of tumour-bearing rats and the incidence of mammary tumours, lymphomas and other tumours in treated rats were similar to those observed in control animals. No liver-cell tumours were reported (Deichmann et al., 1970).

3.2 Other relevant biological data

(a) Metabolism and storage in animals

When ^{14}C-aldrin was administered by gavage to male rats, aldrin, dieldrin and unidentified hydrophilic metabolites were excreted in the faeces and urine. When aldrin administration was discontinued, the percentage of aldrin in the faeces decreased and the percentage of dieldrin increased (Ludwig et al., 1964). When ^{14}C-aldrin was administered to male rabbits the major portion of radioactivity was excreted in the urine rather than in the faeces. Eight urinary metabolites were identified (Menzie, 1969).

Conversion of aldrin to dieldrin has also been reported in cattle, pigs, sheep, rats and poultry (Bann et al., 1956).

Male rat liver microsomes convert aldrin more rapidly to its epoxide dieldrin in vitro than do those of females. The conversion can be inhibited by pesticide synergists such as sesamex (Wong & Terriere, 1965).

Exposure of mammals to aldrin results in the deposition of dieldrin in the adipose tissue of the body (Jager, 1970).

(b) Metabolism in man

Blood samples from six aldrin formulators were analyzed for dieldrin and aldrin. Levels of dieldrin found in the plasma ranged from 0.1 to 0.3 ppm and those for aldrin from 0.01 to 0.13 ppm (Mick et al., 1971).

(c) Carcinogenicity of metabolites

See monograph on dieldrin.

3.3 Observations in man

(a) Studies in workers exposed to aldrin

A study was undertaken in 1968 on 233 workers employed in a factory which had been manufacturing aldrin and dieldrin since 1954-1955, endrin since 1957 and telodrin during 1958-1965. Lengths of exposure ranged from 4-13.3 years (average, 7.6 years). One hundred and eighty-one workers were still employed by the same firm at the time of the study, and their average age was 41 years (range, 22-64). Only two deaths had occurred, and one had been caused by stomach cancer (Jager, 1970). The 52 workers who had left the company have been the subject of a subsequent report. Average age at the time of this survey was 47.4 years (range, 29-72), average occupational exposure was 6.6 years (4.0-12.3) and average time since end of exposure was 7.4 years (4.5-16). Only one death was recorded, and this had not been caused by cancer (Versteeg & Jager, 1973).

4. Comments on Data Reported and Evaluation

4.1 Animal data

Aldrin has been tested only by the oral route in rats and mice. The study in mice was considered to be inadequate for evaluation. Studies in rats were negative in two cases and inadequate in two others.

Aldrin is metabolized to dieldrin, so that exposure to aldrin also involves exposure to dieldrin (see monograph on dieldrin).

4.2 Human data

The epidemiological study which was carried out on occupationally exposed workers does not allow any conclusions to be drawn concerning the existence of an excess risk of developing cancer.

Aldrin is metabolized into dieldrin, so that exposure to aldrin also involves exposure to dieldrin (see monograph on dieldrin).

5. References

Anon. (1972) *Chemical Marketing Reporter*, November 27, p.5

Aue, W.A. & Teli, P.M. (1971) Sampling of air pollutants with support-bonded chromatographic phases. *J. Chromat.*, 62, 15

Bann, J.M., DeCino, T.J., Earle, N.W. & Sun, Y.P. (1956) The fate of aldrin and dieldrin in the animal body. *J. agric. Fd Chem.*, 4, 937

Barthel, W.F., Hawthorne, J.C., Ford, J.H., Bolton, G.C., McDowell, L.L., Grissinger, E.H. & Parsons, D.A. (1969) Pesticide residues in sediments of the lower Mississippi river and its tributaries. *Pest. Monit. J.*, 3, 8

BBLF (Biologische Bundesanstalt für Land- und Forstwirtschaft) (1972) *Pflanzenschutzmittel-Verzeichnis*, Merkblatt Nr.1,23. Auflage, April, Braunschweig, Federal Republic of Germany, p.10

Begliomini, A. & Fravolini, A. (1971) Residui di insetticidi nei mangimi. II. Identificazione e dosaggio gas cromatografico di insetticidi clorurati ed esteri fosforici in mangimi composti. *Arch. vet. ital.*, 22, 109

Bradshaw, J.S., Loveridge, E.L., Rippee, K.P., Peterson, J.L., White, D.A., Barton, J.R. & Fuhriman, D.K. (1972) Seasonal variations in residues of chlorinated hydrocarbon pesticides in the water of the Utah Lake drainage system - 1970 and 1971. *Pest. Monit. J.*, 6, 1616

California Department of Agriculture (1972) *Pesticide Use Report, 1971*, Sacramento, pp. 2-3

California Department of Agriculture (1973) *Pesticide Use Report, 1972*, Sacramento, pp. 2-3

Chemical Information Services, Ltd. (1973) *Directory of West European Chemical Producers*, Oceanside, NY

Corneliussen, P.E. (1969) Pesticide residues in total diet samples (IV) *Pest. Monit. J.*, 2, 140

Cummings, J.G. (1966) Pesticides in the total diet. *Res. Rev.*, 16, 30

Davis, K.J. & Fitzhugh, O.G. (1962) Tumorigenic potential of aldrin and dieldrin for mice. *Toxicol. appl. Pharmacol.*, 4, 187

Decker, G.C., Bruce, W.N. & Bigger, J.H. (1965) The accumulation and dissipation of residues resulting from the use of aldrin in soils. *J. econ. Entomol.*, 58, 266

Deichmann, W.B., Keplinger, M., Sala, F. & Glass, E. (1967) Synergism among oral carcinogens. IV. The simultaneous feeding of four tumorigens to rats. Toxicol. appl. Pharmacol., 11, 88

Deichmann, W.B., MacDonald, W.E., Blum, E., Bevilacqua, M., Radomski, J.L., Keplinger, M. & Balkus, M. (1970) Tumorigenicity of aldrin, dieldrin and endrin in the albino rat. Industr. Med. Surg., 39, 426

Duggan, R.E. (1967) Chlorinated pesticide residues in fluid milk and other dairy products in the United States. Pest. Monit. J., 1, iii, 2

Duggan, R.E. & Corneliussen, P.E. (1972) Dietary intake of pesticide chemicals in the United States (III), June 1968-April 1970. Pest. Monit. J., 5, 331

Duggan, R.E. & Lipscomb, G.Q. (1969) Dietary intake of pesticide chemicals in the United States (II), June 1966-April 1968. Pest. Monit. J., 2, 153

Duggan, R.E., Barry, H.C. & Johnson, L.Y. (1966) Pesticide residues in total diet samples. Science, 151, 101

Duggan, R.E., Barry, H.C. & Johnson, L.Y. (1967) Pesticide residues in total diet samples (II). Pest. Monit. J., 1, ii, 2

Elgar, K.E. (1966) Analysis of crops and soils for residues of soil insecticides aldrin and 'telodrin'. J. Sci. Fd Agric., 17, 541

FAO (1972) FAO Production Yearbook - 1971, 25, Rome, pp. 503-504

FAO/WHO (1967) Evaluation of some pesticide residues in food. FAO/PL: CP/15; WHO/Food Add./67.32

FAO/WHO (1968) 1967 Evaluation of some pesticide residues in food. FAO/PL: 1967/M/11/1; WHO/Food Add./68.30, p. 9

FAO/WHO (1971) 1970 Evaluation of some pesticide residues in food. FAO/AGP/1970/M/12/1; WHO/Food Add./71.42, p. 198

FAO/WHO (1973) Pesticide residues in food. Report of the 1972 Joint FAO/WHO Meeting. Wld Hlth Org. techn. Rep. Ser., No. 525

Fitzhugh, O.G., Nelson, A.A. & Quaife, M.L. (1964) Chronic oral toxicity of aldrin and dieldrin in rats and dogs. Fd Cosmet. Toxicol., 2, 551

Frear, D.E.H., ed. (1972) Pesticide Handbook - Entoma, 24th ed., State College, Pennsylvania, College Science Publishers, p. 91

Gish, C.D. (1970) Organochlorine insecticide residues in soils and soil invertebrates from agricultural lands. Pest. Monit. J., 3, 241

Hayashi, M. (1971) Residues of agricultural drugs and health of children. Shohni Hoken Kenkyu (Children Hlth Study), 30, 1

Jager, K.W. (1970) Aldrin, dieldrin, endrin and telodrin. An epidemiological and toxicological study of long-term occupational exposure. Amsterdam, London, New York, Elsevier, pp. 60, 121-131

Japan Chemical Week, ed. (1973) Japan Chemical Directory, The Chemical Daily Co. Ltd, Osaka, March, p. 358

Johnson, O. (1972) Pesticides '72. Chemical Week, June 21, p. 40

Lichtenstein, E.P., Myrdal, G.R. & Schulz, K.R. (1964) Effect of formulation and mode of application of aldrin on the loss of aldrin and its epoxide from soils and their translocation into carrots. J. econ. Entomol., 57, 133

Lichtenstein, E.P., Schulz, K.R., Fuhremann, T.W. & Liang, T.T. (1970) Degradation of aldrin and heptachlor in field soils during a ten-year period. Translocation into crops. J. agric. Fd Chem., 18, 100

Ludwig, G., Weis, J. & Korte, F. (1964) Excretion and distribution of aldrin-14C and its metabolites after oral administration for a long period of time. Life Sci., 3, 123

Martin, R.J. & Duggan, R.E. (1968) Pesticide residues in total diet samples (III). Pest. Monit. J., 1, iv, 11

McCaskill, W.R., Phillips, B.H., Jr & Thomas, C.A. (1970) Residues of chlorinated hydrocarbons in soybean seed and surface soils from selected counties of South Carolina. Pest. Monit. J., 4, 42

Melnikov, N.N. & Shevchenko, M.G. (1971) Hygienic normalization of pesticide residues and their tolerance levels in foodstuffs in the USSR. Res. Rev., 35, 1

Menzie, C.M. (1969) Aldrin, dieldrin, isodrin, endrin. In: Metabolism of Pesticides, Special Scientific Report - Wildlife, No. 127, Washington DC, US Department of the Interior, p. 24

Mick, D.L., Long, K.R., Dretchen, J.S. & Bonderman, D.P. (1971) Aldrin and dieldrin in human blood components. Arch. environm. Hlth, 23, 177

Mumma, R.O. & Kantner, T.R. (1966) Identification of halogenated pesticides by mass spectroscopy. J. econ. Entomol., 59, 491

Ogata, I. (1972) Merits and demerits of DDT from the viewpoint of sanitation. Gekkan Yakusi (Pharm. Monit.), 14, 1788 (An English abstract is given in Health Aspects of Pesticides Abstract Bulletin No. 730013)

Ragno, M., ed. (1972) *Repertorio Chimico Italiano, Industriale e Commerciale*, Milano, Asiminum

Saha, J.G. & Sumner, A.K. (1971) Organochlorine insecticide residues in soil from vegetable farms in Saskatchewan. *Pest. Monit. J.*, 5, 28

Sand, P.F., Wiersma, G.B. & Landry, J.L. (1972) Pesticide residues in sweet potatoes and soil - 1969. *Pest. Monit. J.*, 5, 342

Seba, D.B. & Corcoran, E.F. (1969) Surface slicks as concentrators of pesticides in the marine environment. *Pest. Monit. J.*, 3, 190

Stanley, C.W., Barney, J.E., II, Helton, M.R. & Yobs, A.R. (1971) Measurement of atmospheric levels of pesticides. *Environm. Sci. Technol.*, 5, 430

Stenersen, J. (1972) Pesticides for plant protection in Norway: legislation, use and residues. *Res. Rev.*, 42, 91

Tabor, E.C. (1966) Contamination of urban air through the use of insecticides. *Trans. N.Y. Acad. Sci.*, 28, 569

Tolle, A., Heeschen, W. & Bluethgen, A. (1972) Chlorierte Insektizide, Fasziolizide und Antibiotika in der Milch. *Ber. Landwirt.*, 50, 720

Trautmann, W.L., Chesters, G. & Pionke, H.B. (1968) Organochlorine insecticide composition of randomly selected soils from nine states 1967. *Pest. Monit. J.*, 2, 93

Treon, J.F. & Cleveland, F.P. (1955) Toxicity of certain chlorinated hydrocarbon insecticides for laboratory animals with special reference to aldrin and dieldrin. *J. agric. Fd Chem.*, 3, 402

UK Ministry of Agriculture, Fisheries & Food (1973) *List of approved products and their uses for farmers and growers*, London, p. 52

US Code of Federal Regulations (1972) Washington DC, US Government Printing Office, 29 CFR 1910.93

US Environmental Protection Agency (1970) *EPA Compendium of Registered Pesticides*, Washington DC, US Government Printing Office, pp. III-A-3.1 - III-A-3.8

US Environmental Protection Agency (1973) Water pollution, prevention and control. Proposed list of toxic pollutants, *US Federal Register*, 38, No. 129, Washington DC, US Government Printing Office, p. 18044

US Tariff Commission (1951) *Synthetic Organic Chemicals, United States Production and Sales, 1950 Second Series, Report No. 173*, Washington DC, US Government Printing Office, p. 127

US Tariff Commission (1968) Imports of Benzenoid Chemicals and Products, 1967, TC Publication 264, Washington DC, US Government Printing Office, p. 85

Versteeg, J.P.J. & Jager, K.W. (1973) Long-term occupational exposure to the insecticides aldrin, dieldrin, endrin and telodrin. Brit. J. industr. Med., 30, 201

Whetstone, R.R. (1964) Chlorocarbons and chlorohydrocarbons: chlorinated derivatives of cyclopentadiene. In: Kirk, R.E. & Othmer, D.F., eds., Encyclopedia of Chemical Technology, 2nd ed., New York, John Wiley & Sons, Vol. 5, p. 240

Wiersma, G.B., Mitchell, W.G. & Stanford, C.L. (1972a) Pesticide residues in onions and soil - 1969. Pest. Monit. J., 5, 345

Wiersma, G.B., Tai, H. & Sand, P.F. (1972b) Pesticide residue levels in soils, FY 1969 - National Soils Monitoring Program. Pest. Monit. J., 6, 194

Wong, D.T. & Terriere, L.C. (1965) Epoxidation of aldrin, isodrin, and heptachlor by rat liver microsomes. Biochem. Pharmacol., 14, 375

ARAMITE[R]

Aramite[R] is a proprietary name for a chemical more properly called 2-(4-<u>tert</u>-butylphenoxy)-1-methylethyl 2-chloroethyl sulphite.

1. Chemical and Physical Data

1.1 Synonyms and trade names

Chem. Abstr. No.: 140-57-8

Aratron; 2-(p-<u>tert</u>-butylphenoxy)isopropyl 2-chloroethyl sulphite; 2-(p-<u>tert</u>-butylphenoxy)isopropyl 2'-chloroethyl sulphite; 2-(p-<u>tert</u>-butylphenoxy)-1-methylethyl 2-chloroethyl ester of sulphurous acid; 2-(p-<u>tert</u>-butylphenoxy)-1-methylethyl 2-chloroethyl sulphite; 2-(p-<u>tert</u>-butylphenoxy)-1-methylethyl 2'-chloroethyl sulphite; 2-(p-<u>tert</u>-butylphenoxy)-1-methylethyl sulphite of 2-chloroethanol; CES; beta-chloroethyl-beta-(p-<u>tert</u>-butylphenoxy)-alpha-methylethyl sulphite; beta-chloroethyl beta'-(p-<u>tert</u>-butylphenoxy)-alpha'-methylethyl sulphite; 2-chloroethyl sulphite of 1-(p-<u>tert</u>-butylphenoxy)-2-propanol; Compound 88R; 2-chloroethyl 1-methyl-2-(p-<u>tert</u>-butylphenoxy)ethyl sulphate; ester of 2-chloroethanol with 2-(p-<u>tert</u>-butylphenoxy)-1-methyl sulphite; Niagaramite; Ortho-Mite

1.2 Chemical formula and molecular weight

$$CH_3-\underset{\underset{CH_3}{|}}{\overset{\overset{CH_3}{|}}{C}}-\underset{}{\bigcirc}-O-CH_2-\underset{\underset{CH_3}{|}}{CH}-O-\overset{\overset{O}{\|}}{S}-O-CH_2CH_2Cl$$

$C_{12}H_{23}ClO_4S$
Mol. wt: 334.9

1.3 Chemical and physical properties of the pure substance

(<u>a</u>) <u>Description</u>: Colourless liquid

(<u>b</u>) <u>Melting-point</u>: -31.7°C

(<u>c</u>) <u>Boiling-point</u>: 175°C at 0.1 mm Hg

(<u>d</u>) <u>Density</u>: 1.145 to 1.162 (techn. product)

(e) <u>Refractive index</u>: n_D^{20} 1.5100 - 1.5118

n_D^{27} 1.5075

(f) <u>Solubility</u>: Practically insoluble in water; miscible with most organic solvents. The solubility in petroleum oils decreases as temperatures are lowered

(g) <u>Volatility</u>: The vapour pressure is <10 mm Hg at 25°C

(h) <u>Stability</u>: In strong sunlight, SO_2 is liberated

(i) <u>Chemical reactivity</u>: Aramite^R hydrolyzes in alkali solutions to form 1-p-<u>tert</u>-butylphenoxypropan-2-ol, ethylene glycol and inorganic sulphite

1.4 Technical products and impurities

The technical product is a dark, amber-coloured liquid which can be sterilized by polypropylene glycol against decomposition by sunlight (Martin, 1971). It may contain 5-10% of bis-2(4-<u>tert</u>-butylphenoxy)-1-methylethyl sulphite (Sternberg et al., 1960).

Aramite^R was formerly available in the United States as a technical grade product containing 90% active ingredient. It was also offered for sale as an 85% emulsifiable concentrate, as a 15% wettable powder and as a 3% active dust (Frear, 1971).

2. Production, Use, Occurrence and Analysis

2.1 Production and use[1]

Commercial production of Aramite^R was first reported in the US in 1950 (US Tariff Commission, 1951); however, the producing company has not reported production of this chemical since 1970. It is believed to have been made by the reaction of 2-chloroethyl chlorosulphinate (made from 2-chloroethanol and thionyl chloride) with 1-(p-<u>tert</u>-butylphenoxy)propanol-2.

---

[1] Data from Chemical Information Services, Stanford Research Institute, USA

Italy was reported to have one producer of Aramite^R in 1973 (Chemical Information Services Ltd., 1973). Aramite^R, earlier registered for use in the US on 39 crops, was registered for use on only 20 crops (all fruits and nuts) as of January 2, 1970; its usage is now restricted to post-harvest applications or on non-bearing trees (US Environmental Protection Agency, 1970).

Although no data are available for total annual US consumption of Aramite^R, it is believed to be quite low. California, a major agricultural state, was reported to have used only 9 thousand kg (36% of this was used on almonds) in 1971 (California Department of Agriculture, 1972) and only 450 kg in 1972 (California Department of Agriculture, 1973).

2.2 Occurrence

No data are available to the Working Group.

2.3 Analysis

Spectrophotometric methods for residue analysis have been published by Brokke et al. (1958) and by Gunther et al. (1951).

Blinn & Gunther (1963) have described a method for distinguishing between Aramite^R and OW-9 (an acaricide consisting of a mixture of two organosulphites closely related in structure to Aramite^R) in citrus fruits using gas chromatography. Archer (1968) has outlined a GLC method for determining Aramite^R in the presence of DDT, toxaphene and endrin in crop residues.

3. Biological Data Relevant to the Evaluation of Carcinogenic Risk to Man

3.1 Carcinogenicity and related studies in animals

(a) Oral administration

Mouse: In both C57BL and C3H strains of mice, groups of 50 males and 50 females were fed diets containing 100, 200 or 400 ppm Aramite^R continuously over 2 years. Controls (100 male and 100 female mice of each strain) received a standard diet. The median survival time was low (48-67 weeks) in C3H mice and higher in C57BL mice (65-74 weeks); however, treated C3H mice showed no higher incidence of mammary or other tumours than did treated C57BL mice. No higher incidence of hepatic or other lesions was reported for the test groups as compared with the controls in both strains of mice (Oser & Oser, 1962).

In a study which was reported as a preliminary note, 18 (C57BL/6 x C3H/Anf)F1 mice of each sex and 18 (C57BL/6 x AKR)F1 mice of each sex were given single doses of 464 mg/kg bw Aramite^R by stomach tube at 7 days of age. The same absolute dose was then given daily until the animals were 28 days of age. Subsequently the animals were fed, *ad libitum*, a diet containing 1112 ppm Aramite^R. Mice were killed at 78-81 weeks. Hepatomas were found in excess over the controls among males of the (C57BL/6 x C3H/Anf)F1 strain, the incidence being 6/16 *versus* 8/79 in the controls. The total tumour incidence in females of the same strain was also increased (Innes et al., 1969).

Rat: Aramite^R was administered at levels of 500, 1580 and 5000 ppm in the diet of groups of 10 male and 10 female FDRL Wistar rats for up to 2 years. Treatment resulted in the development of liver lesions ranging from a single focus of nodular hyperplasia in 1/20 rats receiving 500 ppm, to malignant liver changes in 2/21 rats receiving 1580 ppm, and to liver tumours (diagnosed as hepatomas or cholangiomas) in 6/20 rats receiving 5000 ppm (Oser & Oser, 1960).

In a later study, levels of 100, 200 or 400 ppm Aramite^R were administered in the diet to groups of 50 male and 50 female (Wistar) FDRL, Sprague-Dawley (SD) or Carworth Farm-Nelson (CFN) rats for 2 years. The following liver changes were noted: 2 liver carcinomas and 5 bile duct adenomas in 7/90 FDRL rats fed 400 ppm, with no similar lesions in 193 controls; and bile duct adenomas in 2/93, 1/90 and 2/96 CFN rats receiving the 3 dose levels, respectively, as compared with 0/180 in the controls. Liver lesions were not found in the groups of 41-92 SD rats examined; however, they suffered from respiratory infection, and the medial survival times ranged from 36-55 weeks. The incidence of hyperplastic nodules was increased in the livers of FDRL rats fed 400 ppm and of CFN rats fed 200 and 400 ppm: the respective incidences were 20/90, 10/90 and 22/96 compared with 2/193 in FDRL and 5/180 in CFN controls (Oser & Oser, 1962; Popper et al., 1969).

Groups of 30 male and 30 female Osborne-Mendel rats were administered 200 ppm Aramite^R for 27 months. One haemangioma of the liver was found; no liver tumours occurred in the controls. Tumours at other sites were distributed similarly in the experimental and control groups (Deichmann et al., 1967).

<u>Dog</u>: In a study lasting 3½ years, 17 male and 23 female mongrel dogs were divided into three groups of 12, 12 and 16 animals, which received diets containing 0, 500 or 828-1,420 ppm Aramite^R, respectively. A total of 19 treated dogs died or were killed between 462 and 1,220 days. Of the 5 dogs dying before 811 days, one had neoplastic nodules in the liver. Cancer of the biliary system was found in all of the 14 remaining dogs dying after this time. Of these, adenocarcinomas of both the gall bladder and the extrahepatic biliary ducts occurred in 7 dogs, mainly in those on the higher average dietary concentrations of Aramite^R for the longest periods; 1 dog had carcinoma of both the gall bladder and the intrahepatic biliary ducts; 3 dogs had carcinomas of the extra- and intrahepatic biliary ducts; 2 dogs had adenocarcinomas of the extrahepatic biliary ducts; and 1 dog had a single adenocarcinoma of the gall bladder. There were no calculi present in the gall bladder or the biliary ducts. Five of the 14 dogs had neoplastic liver nodules as well, but no malignant changes were seen in these nodules. Controls remained essentially normal, and tumours did not occur in these animals (Sternberg et al., 1960).

(b) <u>Skin application</u>

<u>Mouse</u>: Two groups of 50 male and 50 female C3H/Anf mice received weekly skin applications of either 0.1 or 10 mg Aramite^R in 0.2 ml acetone. The mean survival times exceeded 400 days, except in females given the lowest dose, for which it was 328 days. The total doses ranged from 0.3-9.0 mg/mouse at the lower dose level and 20-1040 mg/mouse at the higher level. Gross examination revealed no skin tumours; histological examination of the skin was limited to 5-24 mice per group of 50 (Hodge et al., 1966).

(c) Subcutaneous and/or intramuscular administration

Mouse: Aramite^R in trioctanoin was injected subcutaneously into a group of 50 male and 50 female young adult C3H/Anf mice as single doses of 10 mg. The mean survival times were 533 days in the males and 401 days in the females. Gross examination revealed no local tumours; histological examination of the skin was limited to 5 female and to 22 male mice (Hodge et al., 1966).

3.2 Other relevant biological data

No data are available to the Working Group.

3.3 Observations in man

No data are available to the Working Group.

4. Comments on Data Reported and Evaluation[1]

4.1 Animal data

Aramite^R is carcinogenic in the rat and dog following its oral administration. It produced liver tumours in the rat and carcinomas of the gall bladder and biliary ducts in the dog.

Aramite^R was tested in 4 strains of mice by the oral route and produced a significant increase of hepatomas in males of one strain.

No tumours were reported in limited studies involving skin application and subcutaneous injection (single-dose) in mice.

4.2 Human data

No epidemiological studies were available to the Working Group.

---

[1] See also the section "Animal Data in Relation to the Evaluation of Risk to Man" in the introduction to this volume.

5. References

Archer, T.E. (1968) Quantitative measurement of combinations of aramite, DDT, toxaphene and endrin in crop residues. Bull. environm. Contam. Toxicol., 3, 71

Blinn, R.C. & Gunther, F.A. (1963) Procedure for distinguishing compound OW-9 residues from aramite residues on citrus fruits. J. Ass. off. agric. Chem., 46, 204

Brokke, M.E., Kiigemagi, U. & Terriere, L.C. (1958) A spectrophotometric determination of 2-(p-tert-butylphenoxy)-1-methylethyl 2-chloroethyl sulphite (aramite) residues. J. agric. Fd Chem., 6, 26

California Department of Agriculture (1972) Pesticide Use Report, 1971, Sacramento, p. 15

California Department of Agriculture (1973) Pesticide Use Report, 1972, Sacramento, pp. 16-17

Chemical Information Services Ltd. (1973) Directory of West European Chemical Producers, Oceanside, NY

Deichmann, W.B., Keplinger, M., Sala, F. & Glass, E. (1967) Synergism among oral carcinogens. IV. The simultaneous feeding of four tumorigens to rats. Toxicol. appl. Pharmacol., 11, 88

Frear, D.E.H., ed. (1971) Pesticide Handbook - Entoma, 23rd ed., State College, Pennsylvania, College Science Publishers, p. 53

Gunther, F.A., Blinn, R.C., Kolbezen, M.J., Barkley, J.H., Harris, W.D. & Simon, H.S. (1951) Microestimation of 2(p-tert-butylphenoxy)isopropyl-2-chloroethyl sulfite residues. Analyt. Chem., 23, 1835

Hodge, H.C., Maynard, E.A., Downs, W.L., Ashton, J.K. & Salerno, L.L. (1966) Tests on mice for evaluating carcinogenicity. Toxicol. appl. Pharmacol., 9, 583

Innes, J.R.M., Ulland, B.M., Valerio, M.G., Petrucelli, L., Fishbein, L., Hart, E.R., Pallotta, A.J., Bates, R.R., Falk, H.L., Gart, J.J., Klein, M., Mitchell, I. & Peters, J. (1969) Bioassay of pesticides and industrial chemicals for tumorigenicity in mice. A preliminary note. J. nat. Cancer Inst., 42, 1101

Martin, J., ed. (1971) Pesticide Manual. Basic Information on the Chemicals used as Active Components of Pesticides, 2nd ed., Ombersley, British Crop Protection Council, p. 65

Oser, B.L. & Oser, M. (1960) 2-(p-tert-Butylphenoxy)isopropyl 2-chloroethyl sulphite (Aramite^R). I. Acute, subacute and chronic oral toxicity. Toxicol. appl. Pharmacol., 2, 441

Oser, B.L. & Oser, M. (1962) 2-(p-tert-Butylphenoxy)isopropyl 2-chloroethyl sulphite (Aramite^R). II. Carcinogenicity. Toxicol. appl. Pharmacol., 4, 70

Popper, H., Sternberg, S.S., Oser, B.L. & Oser, M. (1960) The carcinogenic effect of aramite in rats. A study of hepatic nodules. Cancer, 13, 1035

Sternberg, S.S., Popper, H., Oser, B.L. & Oser, M. (1960) Gallbladder and bile duct adenocarcinomas in dogs after long term feeding of aramite. Cancer, 13, 780

US Environmental Protection Agency (1970) EPA Compendium of Registered Pesticides, Volume III, Insecticides, Acaricides, Moluscicides and Antifouling Compounds, Washington DC, US Government Printing Office, p. III-B-26

US Tariff Commission (1951) Synthetic Organic Chemicals, United States Production and Sales, 1950 Second Series, Report No. 173, Washington DC, US Government Printing Office, p. 127

BHC(TECHNICAL GRADES) AND LINDANE

BHC is the common name approved by the International Standards Organization for the mixed isomers of 1,2,3,4,5,6-hexachlorocyclohexane. A review on these compounds is available (FAO/WHO, 1969).

Lindane is the common name approved by the International Standards Organization (except in the United Kingdom) for the gamma-isomer of 1,2,3,4,5,6-hexachlorocyclohexane. Several reviews on this compound are available (FAO/WHO, 1967, 1968, 1969, 1970).

1. Chemical and Physical Data

1.1 Synonyms and trade names

(a) BHC (Technical grades)

Mixture of isomers

Chem. Abstr. Nos: 608-73-1 and MX 800-74-29

666; benzene hexachloride*; DBH; Gammexane; HCCH; HCH; Hexa; hexachlorocyclohexane; 1,2,3,4,5,6-hexachlorocyclohexane; Hexachlor; Hexyclan

alpha-Isomer

Chem. Abstr. No.: 319-84-6

alpha-Benzene hexachloride; alpha-BHC; alpha-HCH; 1,2,3,4,5,6-hexachloro-alpha-cyclohexane; alpha-hexachlorocyclohexane; 1,2,3,4,5,6-hexachlorocyclohexane, alpha-isomer; alpha-lindane

beta-Isomer

Chem. Abstr. No.: 319-85-7

trans-alpha-Benzene hexachloride; beta-benzene hexachloride;

---

* Some sources feel that the name benzene hexachloride should not be used for BHC, since it may be confused with hexachlorobenzene, which is a different chemical (Chem. Abstr. No.: 118-74-1).

beta-BHC; 1,2,3,4,5,6-hexachloro-beta-cyclohexane; 1,2,3,4,5,6-hexachloro-<u>trans</u>-cyclohexane; beta-hexachlorocyclohexane; beta-1,2,3,4,5,6-hexachlorocyclohexane; 1,2,3,4,5,6,-hexachlorocyclohexane, beta-isomer; beta-lindane

<u>gamma-Isomer</u>

Chem. Abstr. No.: 58-89-9
(See lindane)

<u>delta-Isomer</u>

Chem. Abstr. No.: 319-86-8

delta-Benzene hexachloride; delta-BHC; delta-HCH; 1,2,3,4,5,6-hexachlorocyclohexane; delta-1,2,3,4,5,6-hexachlorocyclohexane; 1,2,3,4,5,6-hexachlorocyclohexane, delta-isomer; delta-lindane

<u>epsilon-Isomer</u>

Chem. Abstr. No.: 610-81-07

epsilon-Benzene hexachloride; epsilon-BHC; epsilon-HCH; 1,2,3,4,5,6-hexachloro-epsilon cyclohexane; epsilon-hexachlorocyclohexane; epsilon-1,2,3,4,5,6-hexachlorocyclohexane; 1,2,3,4,5,6-hexachlorocyclohexane, epsilon-isomer; epsilon-lindane

<u>zeta-Isomer</u>

Chem. Abstr. No.: 610-81-18

zeta-HCH; 1,2,3,4,5,6-hexachlorocyclohexane, zeta-isomer; zeta-lindane

<u>eta-Isomer</u>

Chem. Abstr. No.: 610-81-29

eta-HCH; 1,2,3,4,5,6-hexachlorocyclohexane, eta-isomer; eta-lindane

<u>theta-Isomer</u>

Chem. Abstr. No.: 610-81-30

theta-HCH; 1,2,3,4,5,6-hexachlorocyclohexane, theta-isomer; theta-lindane

(b) Lindane

Aficide; Agrisol G-20; Agrocide; Aparasin; Aphtiria; Ben-Hex; Bexol; Detox 25; ENT 7,796; gamma-benzene hexachloride; gamma-BHC; gamma-HCH; gamma-hexachlorocyclohexane; gamma-1,2,3,4,5,6-hexachlorocyclohexane; Gammahexa; Gammahexane; gamma-isomer of benzene hexachloride; gamma-isomer of 1,2,3,4,5,6-hexachlorocyclohexane; gamma-lindane; Gammexane; Gexane; Hexachloran; Hexachlorane; 1,2,3,4,5,6-hexachlorocyclohexane, gamma-isomer; Jacutin; Kwell; Lorexane; Streunex; Tri-6

1.2 Chemical formula and molecular weight

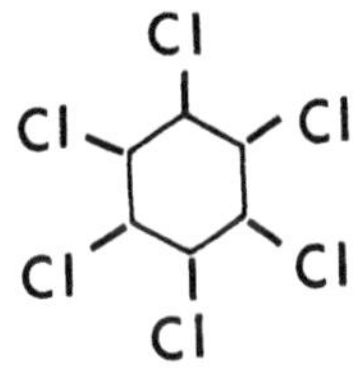

$C_6H_6Cl_6$ Mol. wt: 290.9

Isomers differ in spatial positions of the chlorine atoms on the boat and chair forms

1.3 Chemical and physical properties of the pure substances

α-Isomer

(a) Description: Colourless, crystalline solid with a persistent, acrid odour

(b) Melting-point: 158°C

(c) Solubility: Practically insoluble in water; readily soluble in chloroform and in benzene

(d) Volatility: Vapour pressure is 0.06 mm Hg at 40°C; volatile with steam

β-Isomer

(a) Description: Colourless, crystalline solid

(b) Melting-point: 312°C

(c) Solubility: Slightly soluble in chloroform and in benzene; very slightly soluble in water

(d) Volatility: Vapour pressure is 0.17 mm Hg at 40°C; not volatile with steam

γ-Isomer

(a) Description: Colourless, crystalline solid

(b) Melting-point: 112.5°C

(c) Solubility: Very soluble in chloroform, ethanol, acetone, ether and benzene. Solubility is about 10 mg/l in water

(d) Volatility: Vapour pressure is 0.14 mm Hg at 40°C

(e) Chemical reactivity: With the exception of the β-isomer, the isomers of BHC are dehydrochlorinated by alkalis, mainly to 1,2,4-trichlorobenzene. The δ- and ε-isomers yield, in addition, lesser quantities of 1,2,3-and 1,3,5-trichlorobenzenes (Hardie, 1964).

1.4 Technical products and impurities

(a) BHC (Technical grades)

Technical BHC is a brownish-to-white, crystalline substance (mp 65°C) with a penetrating, musty odour reminiscent of that of phosgene. The content of the isomers in technical BHC varies depending on the manufacturing conditions. An example of the range of isomers follows: α-isomer, 55-70%; β-isomer, 6-8%; γ-isomer, 10-18%; δ-isomer, 3-4%; ε-isomer, very small amounts (Hardie, 1964). In addition, the crude product may contain varying quantities of chlorine-substitution derivatives of cyclohexene and benzene (Stijve & Cardinale, 1972). Technical grades of BHC are formulated as emulsifiable concentrates, wettable powders and dusts.

(b) Lindane

Technical products called "lindane", containing at least 99% of the γ-isomer, are available in many countries. These are formulated into emulsifiable concentrates, wettable powders, dusts, crystals and into solids for smoke generators and thermal vaporizers.

2. Production, Use, Occurrence & Analysis

2.1 Production and use[1]

(a) <u>BHC (Technical grades)</u>

BHC was first synthesized in 1825, but it was not until 1941-1942 that its insecticidal properties were discovered in both England and France. Commercial production of BHC was first reported in the United States in 1945 (US Tariff Commission, 1946). The chlorination of benzene in the presence of ultraviolet light produces a mixture of isomers, which is normally used only as the intermediate for the production of mixtures with higher concentrations of the γ-isomer (Hardie, 1964).

US production of BHC reached a maximum in 1951, when 16 companies produced 53 million kg containing 8 million kg of the γ-isomer (US Tariff Commission, 1952). By 1963, the last year for which production data were reported, the number of producers had dropped to five, and total combined US production of BHC and the pure γ-isomer (lindane) amounted to less than 3 million kg, the amount of γ-isomer being equivalent to 0.8 million kg (US Tariff Commission, 1964). About 3 million kg of BHC were sold in 1967 (US Tariff Commission, 1969), and in 1971 only one US company was still producing this chemical (Stanford Research Institute, 1972).

The following European countries were reported to be producing BHC (technical grades) in 1973 (number of producing companies is given in parentheses): Federal Republic of Germany (1), France (1) and Italy (2) (Economic Documentation Office, 1973). One company in the United Kingdom may also be producing BHC (technical grades).

Imports of this material by European countries in 1971 were reported to have been as follows (thousand kg): Belgium, Luxembourg (319); Federal Republic of Germany (215); France (42); Italy (764); and The Netherlands (225). Exports of this material by European countries in 1971

---

[1] Data from Chemical Information Services, Stanford Research Institute, USA

were reported to have been as follows (thousand kg): Federal Republic of Germany (1729); France (938); Italy (41); and the Netherlands (6) (European Economic Community, 1972).

Production of BHC was prohibited in Japan in 1970, and restrictions were placed on its agricultural use (Anon, 1970); thus, Japanese deliveries of BHC dust in 1971 totalled only 1.2 million kg (Chemical Daily Co., 1972), and the production of BHC was reduced from 35.4 million kg in 1969 to only 2 million kg in 1970 (Hayashi, 1971).

In 1969, Brazilian production of BHC was reported to have been 6.8 million kg, up from 2.7 million kg in 1965 (US Department of Commerce, 1972).

BHC production began in India in 1953, and by 1968 there were 3 producers with an estimated combined production of 11.5 million kg. In the fiscal year 1969 imports into India amounted to 1 million kg (US Department of Commerce, 1970).

The only known use of BHC is as an insecticide. In its early years, it was widely used against the cotton boll-weevil but was subsequently displaced from this market by other pesticides. In recent years, it has been used primarily against insect attack on structures.

As of March 27, 1970 technical BHC was approved in the US for use on 62 agricultural crops (including several types of seeds), with tolerances for residues on raw agricultural commodities set at 1 ppm and with restrictions on the use of treated seeds. It was also approved for use as an insecticide on hogs and on uncultivated land and for the control of outdoor insects (US Environmental Protection Agency, 1970).

BHC usage in California, a major agricultural state, was reported to have been 1,270 kg in 1971 (California Department of Agriculture, 1972) and 950 kg (over 80% of this was for control of insects in residences) in 1972 (California Department of Agriculture, 1973).

Annual world-wide use of BHC was estimated in 1968 to have been 54-64 million kg, including 4.6-5.4 million kg of lindane (FAO/WHO, 1969).

In Austria, this material is not approved for use in the treatment of foods or animal feeds; the Federal Republic of Germany, however, permits

its use in the control of biting insects and for seed treatment. Technical grades of BHC are not approved for use as plant protection agents in Switzerland (EFOWG; EFLP; SFRA, 1972); however, in the United Kingdom technical BHC is approved for use in agriculture in certain specified situations such as dusts, sprays and smokes (UK Ministry of Agriculture, Fisheries and Food, 1973).

(b) Lindane

It was not until 1944 that the insecticidal properties of crude BHC were found to be due entirely to the γ-isomer (Hardie, 1964). Methods were subsequently developed for isolating high purity γ-isomer, and commercial production of lindane was first reported in the US in 1950 (US Tariff Commission, 1951). Lindane is produced commercially by selective crystallization of crude BHC (Spencer, 1968).

It is believed that the quantity of lindane produced in the US probably reached a maximum in the early 1950's and fell rapidly thereafter; only one US company has reported production since 1956. US production has been estimated to have been 500 thousand kg in 1964 (Hardie, 1964) and to have been less than this in 1971 (Johnson, 1972). Imports of lindane through the principal US customs districts were reported to have been 60 thousand kg in 1972 (US Tariff Commission, 1973).

Japan produced 1.3 million kg lindane in 1970 (Hayashi, 1971).

The following European countries were reported to be producing lindane in 1973 (number of producing companies given in parentheses): Federal Republic of Germany (2), France (5), Italy (3), Spain (2), United Kingdom (1, and another company is also believed to be in production) (Chemical Information Services Ltd, 1973; Economic Documentation Office, 1973). In 1970, The Netherlands was reported to have imported 251 thousand kg of lindane (US Department of Commerce, 1972).

India is reported to have commissioned the construction of a lindane plant to help meet its 100 thousand kg/year requirements (Anon., 1972).

The only known use of lindane is as an insecticide. In recent years, its major use is believed to be against insect attack on residential and other structures. A very small amount of lindane is believed to be used in human medicine as a scabicide.

As of April 6, 1973 lindane was approved in the US for use on 67 agricultural crops (including several types of seeds) and in water used in transplanting 24 vegetables and tobacco. Tolerances for residues on raw agricultural commodities were set at 1-3 ppm, and restrictions were in effect on the use of treated seeds. It was also approved for insecticidal uses: (1) on beef cattle, hogs, goats and sheep; (2) in barns, feed rooms and empty grain bins (excluding poultry houses, dairy barns and milk rooms); (3) on uncultivated land; and (4) for control of outdoor insects (US Environmental Protection Agency, 1973).

Lindane usage in California, a major agricultural state, was reported to have been 4.2 thousand kg in 1971 (California Department of Agriculture, 1972) and 5.4 thousand kg in 1972 (42% was for control of insects in residences and 33% for control of insects in other structures) (California Department of Agriculture, 1973).

Annual world-wide use of lindane was estimated in 1968 to have been 4.5-5.4 million kg (FAO/WHO, 1969). Morrison (1972) reported that the use of lindane is banned in Sweden and in Finland, and that it is subject to limitations in Canada. In Austria, this material may not be used for the treatment of foods or animal feeds, and in the Federal Republic of Germany it is not permitted to be used on wheat supplies and derived products but is allowed in a number of agricultural applications (BBLF, 1972). In Portugal, lindane is authorized for sale alone or in combination with several pesticides (Chaby Nunes & Oliveira Nobre, 1972), and in Switzerland it is approved for use in controlling a variety of insects (EFOWG; EFLP; SFRA, 1972). Lindane is also widely used in the United Kingdom (UK Ministry of Agriculture, Fisheries and Food, 1973). In Kenya and other African countries, it continues to be used as a dry bean protectant (WHO, 1972).

An indication of possible uses of lindane can be derived from the FAO/WHO recommended residue limits for that substance in the following food products: vegetables, cranberries, cherries, grapes, plums, strawberries, beans (dried), raw cereals and fat of meat from cattle, pigs and sheep, milk and milk products, poultry and eggs (yolk) (FAO/WHO, 1973).

2.2 Occurrence

(a) Occupational exposure

During forest spraying the mean concentration of BHC in the air ranged from 3.2-48.4 mg/m^3 and the dermal exposure from 0.03-0.06 mg/cm^2/hr, depending on the location of sampling. From this, a respiratory exposure of 0.35-5.59 mg/kg bw/8 hrs and a dermal exposure of 7.40-38.82 mg/kg bw/8 hrs were calculated (Wassermann et al., 1960). During cropland spraying concentrations in the air ranged from 0.1-2 mg/m^3 (Kale & Dangwal, 1971).

(b) Air and rain

Average concentrations in nine localities in various parts of the US ranged from 0.4-1.4 ng/m^3 for lindane and from 0.7-5.0 ng/m^3 for α-BHC. Maximum levels were 2.2 ng/m^3 (β-BHC), 7.0 ng/m^3 (lindane) and 9.9 ng/m^3 (α-BHC, δ-BHC) (Stanley et al., 1971). In urban air in Japan 54 ng/m^3 have been detected (Wakimoto et al., 1970); and very small quantities (1 g α-BHC/10^{12} g air and 5 g lindane/10^{12} g air) have been found in London and suburbs (Abbott et al., 1966).

In rainwater, average concentrations of 23 ng/l for α-BHC (Abbott et al., 1965) and 5-100 ng/l for lindane have been found (Abbott et al., 1965; Bevenue et al., 1972; Cohen & Pinkerton, 1966; Tarrant & Tatton, 1968; Wheatley & Hardman, 1965).

(c) Soil and water

Lindane disappears relatively rapidly from treated soils, especially from moist soils, compared to other organochlorine insecticides, due to a combination of factors: smaller applications are needed; and it has a higher water solubility, faster evaporation and lesser absorption by organic matter (WHO, 1972). In 13 of 41 soil samples concentrations ranged from 0.001-0.005 ppm γ-BHC (Trautmann et al., 1986); and in other soil samples, from 0.01-0.35 ppm lindane (mean value, 0.01 ppm) have been found (Saha & Sumner, 1971; Wiersma et al., 1972). Of 117.3 kg/ha BHC added to soil during 1950-53, 7.7% remained in 1968 (Chisholm & MacPhee, 1972).

Small amounts of lindane (0.2 ng/l) have also been reported in drinking-water in Hawaii (Bevenue et al., 1972). Concentrations of lindane in surface water in the US ranged from 0-0.02 µg/l (Brown & Nishioka, 1967; Lichtenberg et al., 1970; Manigold & Schulze, 1969), lindane being present in about 15% of the samples (Lichtenberg et al., 1970). In the Federal Republic of Germany lindane was present in all samples taken, in concentrations ranging from 0.005-7.1 µg/l, while α-BHC was present in about 70% of the samples, in concentrations ranging from 0.005-2.4 µg/l (Herzel, 1972).

(d) *Animals and plants*

BHC is stored in the adipose tissue, liver, brain and muscle of mammals, fish, reptiles and birds and in algae and plankton. In fatty tissue of fish, concentrations ranged from <0.01-0.59 ppm lindane (Hannon et al., 1970) and in whole fish, from 0.01-4.37 ppm total BHC, with a median level of approximately 0.02 ppm (Henderson et al., 1971). In oysters, a median value of 0.01 ppm BHC-lindane was found in 55 of 133 samples (Bugg et al., 1967). In the livers of Antarctic penguins mean concentrations ranged from 0.002-0.008 ppm β-BHC and from 0-0.003 ppm γ-BHC (Tatton & Ruzicka, 1967). In wild birds, maximum values of 0.4 ppm γ-BHC and 6 ppm other BHC isomers were found in brain (Walker et al., 1967), and Martin & Nickerson (1972) detected from 0.005-0.39 ppm BHC in all of 125 starlings examined. In 4 of 48 pheasants, 0.04 ppm (fat and brain) and 0.01 ppm (brain) lindane could be detected (Linder & Dahlgren, 1970). Greichus et al. (1968) found no more than 0.01 ppm lindane in the fat of 75% of pheasants examined.

(e) *Food*

In the US, the UK and Japan several analyses of total diets have been carried out (Abbott et al., 1969; Corneliussen, 1969, 1970, 1972; Cummings, 1966; Duggan & Corneliussen, 1972; Duggan & Lipscomb, 1969; Duggan & Weatherwax, 1967; Duggan et al., 1966, 1967, 1971; Egan et al., 1966; Kojima, 1972; Martin & Duggan, 1968; McGill & Robinson, 1968; Uyeta et al., 1971). A slight decline in dietary levels of lindane and an almost stable value for dietary levels of BHC have been found for the years 1965-1970 (Duggan & Corneliussen, 1972).

In meat, fish and poultry, the maximum values of BHC ranged from 0.05

ppm (Cummings, 1966) to 0.2 ppm (Corneliussen, 1972; Martin & Duggan, 1968), and the maximum value of lindane from 0.03 ppm (Corneliussen, 1969, 1970) to 0.08 ppm (Corneliussen, 1972). The Joint FAO/WHO Meetings (FAO/WHO, 1967, 1969) summarized the data on the controlled use of lindane in poultry houses, for spraying cattle and in feeding studies in poultry. In hens receiving 0.1, 1.0 and 10 ppm lindane in their diets for 60 days, residues in egg yolks were 0.26, 0.46 and 4.96 ppm, respectively (Ware & Naber, 1961). After feeding poultry at levels of 4, 16 and 64 ppm for 27 days, Harrison et al. (1963) found 19.1, 56.4 and 156.0 ppm, respectively, in the body fat.

BHC occurs in dairy products mostly from feed, and more α- or β-BHC than lindane is generally found. Williams et al. (1964) found 0.002, 0.006 and 0.015 ppm lindane residues in the milk of cows fed 0.05, 0.15 and 0.30 ppm, respectively, of lindane in their daily ration for 35 days. Residue levels for α-BHC were as much as 0.15 ppm (Bro-Rasmussen et al., 1968; Duggan, 1967; Frank et al., 1970; Tolle, 1972). In Japan, an average of 0.01-1.1 ppm total BHC (mostly the β-isomer) was found in milk (Narafu, 1971), but maximum values of 2.03 ppm β-BHC found in 1970 had declined to 0.17 ppm by 1971 (Kojima, 1972). Uhnak (1971) found as much as 0.8 ppm BHC in milk fat. In total diet studies in the US concentrations of BHC in dairy products ranged from 0.03-0.39 ppm (Corneliussen, 1969, 1970, 1972; Martin & Duggan, 1968).

In human milk, 0.001-0.03 ppm lindane have been detected (Acker & Schulte, 1970; Heyndrickx & Maes, 1969), and the total BHC concentration ranged from <0.0001-0.4 ppm (Curley & Kimbrough, 1969; Egan et al., 1965; Narafu, 1971). Kroger (1972) detected 0.08 ppm in human milk fat.

Usually only small amounts have been detected in fruits and vegetables. Maximum values found in different vegetables ranged from 0.006 ppm lindane (Corneliussen, 1969) to 0.015 ppm BHC and/or lindane (Cummings, 1966), and in garden fruits from 0.003 ppm lindane (Corneliussen, 1972), to 0.025 ppm (Duggan et al., 1966) have been found. Small amounts have also been detected in oils and fats (up to 0.04 ppm BHC), in grains and cereals (up to 0.03 ppm lindane) and in sugars (up to 0.02 ppm BHC and/or lindane) (Corneliussen, 1969, 1970; Cummings, 1966).

In the US the total dietary intake of lindane was 4 μg/man/day in 1965 and 1966, 5 μg/man/day in 1967, 3 μg/man/day in 1968 and 1 μg in 1969 and 1970; and for BHC, 4 μg/man/day in 1966, 3 μg/man/day in 1968, 2 μg/man/day in 1965 and 1967 and 1 μg/man/day in 1969 and 1970 (Duggan & Corneliussen, 1972). This amounts to a 6-year average of 0.03 μg/kg bw/day for BHC and of 0.05 μg/kg bw/day for lindane (Duggan & Corneliussen, 1972).

Similar investigations in the UK indicate an average total BHC intake, including lindane, of 0.2 μg/kg bw/day (Abbott et al., 1969) and 0.14 μg/kg bw/day (Department of Trade & Industry, 1973). In Japan, an intake of 0.63-1.34 μg/kg bw/day has been estimated (Kojima, 1972; Uyeta et al., 1971). The acceptable daily intake (ADI) of lindane has been set at 12.5 μg/kg bw/day (WHO, 1972); no ADI has yet been set for technical BHC because of variations in composition of the material used.

A threshold limit value of 0.5 mg/m^3 has been established for an 8-hour time-weighted average occupational exposure in the US (US Code of Federal Regulations, 1972).

2.3 Analysis

A general approach to the analysis of organochlorine pesticides has been given in the preamble (p. 16). The quantitative gas chromatographic determination of α-, β-, γ-, δ-, ε-, and η-BHC isomers, together with γ- and ε-heptachlorocyclohexanes, has been described by Davis & Joseph (1967), and a rapid method for the separation of the five main isomers and for the quantitative determination of lindane is given by Trombetti & Gordini (1971).

A gas chromatographic method for milk fat is described by Szokolay et al. (1971) and a thin-layer chromatographic method for determination in air and food by Uporova & Shtyler (1971 a & b).

3. Biological Data Relevant to the Evaluation of Carcinogenic Risk to Man

3.1 Carcinogenicity and related studies in animals

(a) Oral administration

Mouse: Three groups of 20 male dd mice were fed for 24 weeks on diets containing either 6.6, 66.0 or 660 ppm technical BHC, the composition of which was: 66.6% α-isomer, 11.3% β-isomer, 15.2% γ-isomer, 6.3% δ-isomer, 0.6% others. All mice were killed after 24 weeks. Hepatomas were found in 20/20 animals fed 660 ppm technical BHC, but no such tumours were observed in mice receiving the lower doses. No nodules or tumours occurred in 14 male controls (the spontaneous incidence of liver tumours in this strain of mice is very low) (Nagasaki et al., 1971, 1972a).

In a subsequent experiment reported in a preliminary communication, groups of 20 male dd mice were fed the α, β, γ or δ isomers separately, each at concentrations of 100, 250 or 500 ppm. The experiment was terminated at 24 weeks. Multiple liver tumours, up to 2.0 cm in diameter, were found in all animals given 500 ppm α-BHC, while nodules up to 0.3 cm in diameter were found in 9/20 mice given 250 ppm α-BHC; no lesions were found in mice given 100 ppm α-BHC. No tumours were produced with any dose level of the other three isomers nor in a similar group of 20 controls (Nagasaki et al., 1972b).

In a recent experiment lasting 110 weeks a group of 30 male and 30 female CF1 mice was fed on a diet containing 200 ppm β-BHC, and a group of 29 males and 29 females received a diet containing 400 ppm γ-BHC. A group of controls comprising 44 female and 45 male mice was fed on standard diet. The percentages of animals receiving control 200 ppm β-BHC or 400 ppm γ-BHC diets which bore liver tumours were 24%, 73% and 93%, respectively, in males and 23%, 43% and 69%, respectively, in females. Lung metastases were found in some male animals receiving β- and γ-BHC and in some females receiving γ-BHC. The incidence of other tumours was not increased by exposure to either isomer (Thorpe & Walker, 1973).

In a study reported while the experiment was still in progress, groups of 20 male ICR-JCL mice aged 5 weeks were fed on a diet containing 600 ppm technical BHC, pure α-, β- or γ-isomers or a mixture of δ + ε-BHC. Further groups of 20 mice received a control diet or one containing 300 ppm γ-BHC. Gross examination of 10 animals of each group after 26 weeks showed liver nodules to be present in those receiving 600 ppm technical BHC, α-BHC, γ-BHC and the δ + ε mixture. Histologically benign liver tumours were observed in all treated groups except in the group receiving 300 ppm γ-BHC. In animals administered diets containing α-BHC and the δ + ε mixture, the histological appearance of tumours was frequently malignant (Goto et al., 1972).

Rat: Groups of 10 male and 10 female rats were fed for their lifespan on diets containing 10, 50, 100 or 800 ppm technical BHC; 10, 50, 100 or 800 ppm α-BHC; 10, 100 or 800 ppm β-BHC; 5, 10, 50, 100, 400, 800 or 1600 ppm γ-BHC as a solution in oil; or 10, 100 or 800 ppm powdered γ-BHC. Technical BHC contained 64% α-, 10% β-, 13% γ-, 9% δ- and 1.3% ε-isomers. The average lifespan was significantly reduced when all compounds were given at 800 ppm and higher levels. The mean age at death was 58 weeks in a group of 40 control animals and 33-70 weeks in experimental groups; however, the tumour incidence in animals receiving treatment was not greater than in controls. In only 238 animals were the organs examined microscopically (Fitzhugh et al., 1950).

In a further experiment in which rats received diets containing 25, 50 or 100 ppm γ-BHC for 2 years, no significant increase in tumour incidence was observed (Truhaut, 1954).

(b) Skin application

Mouse: A group of 30 stock mice was given twice-weekly applications of a 0.5% solution of γ-BHC in acetone to the skin for 15 months. Twenty-one mice were alive at the end of the treatment, and no skin tumours were produced. One mammary carcinoma and one leukaemia were observed and were considered to be spontaneous (Orr, 1948).

(c) Subcutaneous and/or intramuscular administration

Mouse: In an experiment lasting 10 months no tumours were observed in 12/20 stock mice surviving within this time after s.c. implantations of a paraffin wax pellet containing 3% γ-BHC (Orr, 1948).

3.2 Other relevant biological data

(a) Metabolism and storage in animals

When single doses of ^{36}Cl-labelled α-BHC and γ-BHC were given intra-peritoneally to rats at levels of 200 mg/kg bw and 40 mg/kg bw, respectively, approximately 80% of the total radioactivity was excreted in the urine and 20% in the faeces (Koransky et al., 1964). When labelled β-BHC (unspecified) was administered orally to female Sprague-Dawley rats 80% was found to have been absorbed from the gastro-intestinal tract (Oshiba, 1972).

After intraperitoneal administration of γ-BHC to rats, Grover & Sims (1965) identified 2,3,5- and 2,4,5-trichlorophenol in the urine, either free or as conjugates of glucuronic and/or sulphuric acid possibly resulting from 1,2,4-trichlorobenzene. When weanling Sprague-Dawley rats were fed 400 ppm γ-BHC, 3,4-dichlorophenol, 2,4,6-trichlorophenol, 2,3,4,5- and 2,3,4,6-tetrachlorophenol and 2,3,4,5,6-pentachloro-2-cyclohexen-1-ol were identified in the urine (Chadwick & Freal, 1972).

Davidow & Frawley (1951) fed 800 ppm α- and δ-BHC and 100 ppm β-isomer to rats for 20 months. At the end of the study 3500 ppm α-isomer and 550 ppm δ-isomer were found in the adipose tissue; the levels in other tissues were lower, roughly by about a factor of 10. β-BHC fed at 100 ppm was stored to a greater extent, the concentration in adipose tissue being 1900 ppm; brain contained 130 ppm and liver only 20 ppm. Upon cessation of the dietary exposure to these BHC-isomers, α- and δ-isomers disappeared from the fat depots within three weeks, while the β-isomer persisted in the adipose tissue in small amounts after 14 weeks. The α-, β- and δ-isomers of BHC are also stored in the adipose tissue of dogs, and in this species a considerable amount of the α- and β-isomers is also stored in the adrenals (Davidow & Frawley, 1951).

α, β, γ and δ-BHC were administered separately as an acetone oil solution by stomach tube to Wistar rats at the rate of 50 mg/kg bw daily for 7 days and it was found that the β-isomer was excreted at a slower rate than were the other isomers (Kamada, 1971). Oshiba (1972) found that the deposition of β-BHC in adipose tissue was greater than that of γ-BHC and that when the rats were starved β-BHC was mobilized from the adipose tissue and redistributed. The deposition of γ-BHC in the livers of female Sprague-Dawley rats decreased with an increasing amount of dietary protein (Oshiba & Kawakita, 1972). When α-BHC-^{14}C was given in a single i.p. dose to rats, most of the radioactivity found in the brain was concentrated in areas rich in myelin (Koransky & Ulberg, 1964). In rats fed γ-BHC, this chemical reached equilibrium in adipose tissue within 4-6 weeks, and upon cessation of treatment it disappeared from fat depots within 3 weeks (Davidow & Frawley, 1951). Pretreatment of rats with phenobarbital accelerated the rate of excretion of α- and γ-BHC (Koransky et al., 1964).

(b) Metabolism and storage in man

Following the accidental ingestion of γ-BHC by a 2½ year-old girl, 0.84 ppm and 0.49 ppm γ-BHC were found in the serum 2 hours and 6 hours, respectively, after ingestion. The concentration of γ-BHC in the faeces 24 hours after ingestion was 4,870 ppm. Several urinary metabolites of γ-BHC were identified, i.e., 2,4-dichloro-, 2,4,6-trichloro-, 2,3,5-trichloro- and 2,4,5-trichlorophenols (Starr & Clifford, 1972).

The storage levels of total BHC-isomers in adipose tissue in the general populations of different countries varied from 0.02-1.43 ppm, and the concentrations in human blood ranged from 0.0031-0.0042 ppm (Durham, 1969). Sieper (1972) listed γ-BHC adipose tissue levels in the general population, the lowest concentration being 0.015 ppm in England and the highest that in France, being 1.19 ppm. In 241 human adipose tissue samples from Japan the mean concentration of α-BHC was found to be 0.14 ppm, that of β-BHC 1.28 ppm and that of γ-BHC 0.12 ppm (Curley et al., 1973). Doguchi et al. (1971) found 0.14 ppm α-BHC, 2.92 ppm β-BHC and 0.13 ppm γ-BHC in 21 adipose tissue samples from human females living in metropolitan Tokyo. The total BHC concentration in human adipose tissue samples taken in Budapest averaged 0.76 ppm (Soós et al., 1972); and in Australia, the highest value of total BHC was found to be 2.6 ppm in 75 human adipose tissue samples (Brady & Siyali, 1972).

In a fatal case of γ-BHC poisoning in an 18 month-old infant, about 350 ppm were found in the adipose tissue and 88 ppm in the liver (Joslin et al., 1958).

For additional data on storage, see table in appendix, p. 224.

Trace amounts of total BHC have also been measured in human milk (Curley & Kimbrough, 1969; Tuinstra, 1971), and transplacental passage of α, β, γ-BHC has been found to occur (Curley et al., 1969).

(c) Carcinogenicity of metabolites

Three metabolites, 1,2,4-trichlorobenzene, 2,3,5-trichlorophenol and 2,4,5-trichlorophenol, were administered to groups of 20 male mice for 6 months at a level of 600 ppm in the diet and produced no tumours of the liver in these animals, in contrast to parallel experiments in which the same dose level of BHC isomers (α, β, γ, or the δ + ε mixture) gave rise to benign and/or malignant liver tumours (Goto et al., 1972).

3.3 Observations in man

Chronic liver damage (cirrhosis and chronic hepatitis) has been reported, on the basis of liver biopsy, in 8 workers heavily exposed to BHC, DDT or both for periods ranging from 5-13 years. As far as was feasible, other causes, such as alcoholism, were excluded as the cause of the cirrhosis (Schüttmann, 1968).

In a study on the concentration of chlorinated hydrocarbons in fat and liver of terminal patients, only the more persistent β-isomer of BHC was found. Its concentration in cancer cases did not differ significantly from that found in people dying from infectious or other diseases (Radomski et al., 1968).

Over 30 cases with exposure to BHC or lindane and 21 cases with exposure to BHC and DDT followed by the development of aplastic anaemia have been reported in the literature (Loge, 1965; West, 1967; Woodliff et al., 1966). In addition, the development of leukaemia following lindane exposure has been reported for 2 cases (Jedlicka et al., 1958).

4. Comments on Data Reported and Evaluation[1]

4.1 Animal data

Technical BHC, its pure α-, β- and γ-isomers and the mixture of δ + ε isomers are carcinogenic in mice, producing liver-cell tumours following oral administration. This effect was recorded in both sexes after exposure

---

[1] See also the section "Animal Data in Relation to the Evaluation of Risk to Man" in the introduction to this volume.

to the β- and γ-isomers; the technical compound, the α-isomer and the δ + ε mixture were tested in male mice only.

Available feeding studies in rats were considered inadequate either because survival rates were low, the information reported was insufficient or because the doses given were too low.

No tumours were reported in limited skin application and subcutaneous implantation studies in mice.

4.2 Human data

No epidemiological studies were available to the Working Group. Patients dying with cancer did not show higher concentrations of BHC in fat tissues and liver than did control patients.

No firm conclusions as to a causal relationship with aplastic anaemia and/or leukaemia can be drawn from available case reports.

5. References

Abbott, D.C., Harrison, R.B., Tatton, J.O'G. & Thomson, J. (1965) Organochlorine pesticides in the atmospheric environment. *Nature (Lond.)*, 208, 1317

Abbott, D.C., Holmes, D.C. & Tatton, J.O'G. (1969) Pesticide residues in the total diet in England and Wales 1966-67. II. Organochlorine pesticide residues in the total diet. *J. Sci. Fd Agric.*, 20, 245

Abbott, D.C., Harrison, R.B., Tatton, J.O'G. & Thomson, J. (1966) Organochlorine pesticides in the atmosphere. *Nature (Lond.)*, 211, 259

Acker, Von L. & Schulte, E. (1970) Über das Vorkommen chlorierter Kohlenwasserstoffe im menschlichen Fettgewebe und in Humanmilch. *Dtsch. Lebensmittel-Rundsch.*, 66, 385

Anon. (1970) Use of organochlorine insecticides more restricted by notifications issued by directors general of livestock and agricultural administration bureaus. *Jap. Pest. Inform.*, 3, 22-23 (An English abstract is given in *Health Aspects of Pesticides Abstract Bulletin*, No. 72-2047)

Anon. (1972) *Chemical Industry News - India*, May, p. 35

BBLF (Biologische Bundesanstalt für Land- und Forstwirtschaft) (1972) *Pflanzenschutzmittel-Verzeichnis*, Merkblatt Nr. 1, 23. Auflage, April, Braunschweig, Federal Republic of Germany, pp. 11, 19

Bevenue, A., Hylin, J.W., Kawano, Y. & Kelley, T. (1972) Organochlorine pesticide residues in water, sediment, algae and fish, Hawaii, 1970-71. *Pest. Monit. J.*, 6, 56

Brady, M.N. & Siyali, D.S. (1972) Hexachlorobenzene in human body fat. *Med. J. Austr.*, 1, 158

Bro-Rasmussen, F., Dalgaard-Mikkelsen, Sv., Jakobsen, Th., Koch, Sv.O., Rodin, F., Uhl, E. & Voldum-Clausen, K. (1968) Examinations of Danish milk and butter for contaminating organochlorine insecticides. *Res. Rev.*, 23, 55

Brown, E. & Nishioka, Y.A. (1967) Pesticides in selected western streams - a contribution to the national program. *Pest. Monit. J.*, 1, ii, 38

Bugg, J.C., Jr, Higgins, J.E. & Robertson, E.A., Jr (1967) Chlorinated pesticide levels in the eastern oyster (*Crassostrea virginica*) from selected areas of the South Atlantic and Gulf of Mexico. *Pest. Monit. J.*, 1, iii, 9

California Department of Agriculture (1972) *Pesticide Use Report, 1971*, Sacramento, pp. 24, 102-103

California Department of Agriculture (1973) *Pesticide Use Report, 1972*, Sacramento, pp. 26-27, 113

Chaby Nunes, J. de & Oliveira Nobre, C. de (1972) *Lista dos produtos fitofarmacêuticos com venda autorizada*, Lisbon, Secretaria de Estado da Agricultura, p. 15

Chadwick, R.W. & Freal, J.J. (1972a) The identification of five unreported lindane metabolites recovered from rat urine. *Bull. environm. Contam. Toxicol.*, 7, 137

Chemical Daily Co. (1972) *Japan Chemical Annual*, Tokyo, Mitsui, p. 89

Chemical Information Services, Ltd (1973) *Directory of West European Chemical Producers*, Oceanside, NY

Chisholm, D. & MacPhee, A.W. (1972) Persistence and effects of some pesticides in soil. *J. econ. Entomol.*, 65, 1010

Cohen, J.M. & Pinkerton, C. (1966) Widespread translocation of pesticides by air transport and rainout. *Organic Pesticides in the Environment, Adv. Chem. Ser.*, 60, 163

Corneliussen, P.E. (1969) Pesticide residues in total diet samples (IV). *Pest. Monit. J.*, 2, 140

Corneliussen, P.E. (1970) Pesticide residues in total diet samples (V). *Pest Monit. J.*, 4, 89

Corneliussen, P.E. (1972) Pesticide residues in total diet samples (VI). *Pest. Monit. J.*, 5, 313

Cummings, J.G. (1966) Pesticides in the total diet. *Res. Rev.*, 16, 30

Curley, A. & Kimbrough, R.D. (1969) Chlorinated hydrocarbon insecticides in plasma and milk of pregnant and lactating women. *Arch. environm. Hlth*, 18, 156

Curley, A., Copeland, M.F. & Kimbrough, R.D. (1969) Chlorinated hydrocarbon insecticides in organs of stillborn and blood of newborn babies. *Arch. environm. Hlth*, 19, 628

Curley, A., Burse, V.W., Jennings, R.W., Villanueva, E.C., Tomatis, L. & Akazaki, K. (1973) Chlorinated hydrocarbon pesticides and related compounds in adipose tissue from people of Japan. *Nature (Lond.)*, 242, 338

Davidow, B. & Frawley, J.P. (1951) Tissue distribution, accumulation and elimination of the isomers of benzene hexachloride. *Proc. Soc. exp. Biol. (N.Y.)*, 76, 780

Davis, A. & Joseph, H.M. (1967) Quantitative determination of benzene hexachlorides by gas chromatography. *Analyt. Chem.*, 39, 1016

Department of Trade & Industry (1973) Report of the Government Chemist, 1972, London, HMSO (in press)

Doguchi, M., Ushio, F., Niwayama, K. & Nishida, K. (1971) Pesticide content of human female fat in a metropolitan area of Tokyo. Toritsu Eisei Kenkyusho Kenky Nenpo (Ann. Rep. Tokyo Metrop. Res. Lab. Pub. Hlth), 22, 131

Duggan, R.E. (1967) Chlorinated pesticide residues in fluid milk and other dairy products in the United States. Pest. Monit. J., 1, iii, 2

Duggan, R.E. & Corneliussen, P.E. (1972) Dietary intake of pesticide chemicals in the United States (III), June 1968-April 1970. Pest. Monit. J., 5, 331

Duggan, R.E. & Lipscomb, G.Q. (1969) Dietary intake of pesticide chemicals in the United States (II), June 1966-April 1968. Pest. Monit. J., 2, 153

Duggan, R.E. & Weatherwax, J.R. (1967) Dietary intake of pesticide chemicals. Science, 157, 1006

Duggan, R.E., Barry, H.C. & Johnson, L.Y. (1966) Pesticide residues in total diet samples. Science, 151, 101

Duggan, R.E., Barry, H.C. & Johnson, L.Y. (1967) Pesticide residues in total diet samples (II). Pest. Monit. J., 1, ii, 2

Duggan, R.E., Lipscomb, G.Q., Cox, E.L., Heatwole, R.E. & Kling, R.C. (1971) Pesticide residue levels in foods in the United States from July 1, 1963 to June 30, 1969. Pest. Monit. J., 5, 73

Durham, W.F. (1969) Body burden of pesticides in man. Ann. N.Y. Acad. Sci., 160, 183

Economic Documentation Office (1973) Entoma Europe, 1973-1975, Hilversum, The Netherlands

EFOWG; EFLP; SFRA (Eidg. Forschungsanstalt für Obst-, Wein- und Gartenbau, Wädenswil; Eidg. Forschungsanstalt für landwirtschaftlichen Pflanzenbau, Zürich-Reckenholz; Station fédérale de recherches agronomiques, Lausanne) (1972) Pflanzenschutzmittel-Verzeichnis, Bern, Eidg. Drucksachen- und Materialzentrale, pp. 34-36, 73, 74

Egan, H., Goulding, R., Roburn, J. & Tatton, J.O'G. (1965) Organochlorine pesticide residues in human fat and human milk. Brit. med. J., iii, 66

Egan, H., Holmes, D.C., Roburn, J. & Tatton, J.O'G. (1966) Pesticide residues in foodstuffs in Great Britain. II. Persistent organochlorine pesticide residues in selected foods. J. Sci. Fd Agric., 17, 563

European Economic Community (1972) Foreign Trade, Analytical Tables, Volume C, Chapters 28-38, 1971, Luxembourg, Brussels, Statistical Office of the European Communities

FAO/WHO (1967) Evaluation of some pesticide residues in food. FAO/PL:CP/15; WHO/Food Add./67.32

FAO/WHO (1968) 1967 Evaluations of some pesticide residues in food. FAO/PL: 1967/M/11/1; WHO/Food Add./68.30, p, 9

FAO/WHO (1969) 1968 Evaluations of some pesticide residues in food. FAO/PL/1968/M/9/1; WHO/Food Add./69.35

FAO/WHO (1970) 1969 Evaluations of some pesticide residues in food. FAO/PL/1969/M/17/1; WHO/Food Add./70.38, p. 161

FAO/WHO (1973) Pesticide residues in food. Report of the 1972 Joint FAO/WHO Meeting. Wld Hlth Org. techn. Rep. Ser., No. 525

Fitzhugh, O.G., Nelson, A.A. & Frawley, J.P. (1950) The chronic toxicities of technical benzene hexachloride and its alpha, beta and gamma isomers. J. Pharmacol. exp. Ther., 100, 59

Frank, R., Braun, H.E. & McWade, J.W. (1970) Chlorinated hydrocarbon residues in the milk supply of Ontario, Canada. Pest. Monit. J., 4, 31

Goto, M., Hattori, M., Miyagawa, T. & Enomoto, M. (1972) Beiträge zur ökologischen Chemie. II. Hepatoma-Bildung in Mäusen nach Verabreichung von HCH-Isomeren in hohen Dosen. Chemosphere, 6, 279

Greichus, Y.A., Greichus, A. & Reider, E.G. (1968) Insecticide residues in grouse and pheasant of South Dakota. Pest. Monit. J., 2, 90

Grover, P.L. & Sims, P. (1965) The metabolism of γ-2,3,4,5,6-pentachlorocyclohex-1-ene and γ-hexachlorocyclohexane in rats. Biochem. J., 96, 521

Hannon, M.R., Greichus, Y.A., Applegate, R.L. & Fox, A.C. (1970) Ecological distribution of pesticides in Lake Poinsett, South Dakota. Trans. amer. Fish. Soc., 99, 496

Hardie, D.W.F. (1964) Benzene hexachloride. In: Kirk, R.E. & Othmer, D.F., eds, Encyclopedia of Chemical Technology, 2nd ed., New York, John Wiley & Sons, Vol. 5, pp. 267-281

Harrison, D.L., Poole, W.S.H. & Mol, J.C.M. (1963) Observations on feeding lindane-fortified mash to chickens. N.Z. Vet. J., 11, 137

Hayashi, M. (1971) Residues of agricultural drugs and health of children. Shohni Hoken Kenkyu (Children Hlth Study), 30, 1

Henderson, C., Inglis, A. & Johnson, W.L. (1971) Organochlorine insecticide residues in fish - fall 1969, national pesticide monitoring program. Pest. Monit. J., 5, 1

Herzel, F. (1972) Organochlorine insecticides in surface waters in Germany - 1970 and 1971. Pest. Monit. J., 6, 179

Heyndrickx A. & Maes, R. (1969) The excretion of chlorinated hydrocarbon insecticides in human mother milk. J. Pharm. belg., 24, 459

Jedlička, V.L., Hermanská, Z., Smîda, I. & Kouba, A. (1958) Paramyeloblastic leukaemia appearing simultaneously in two blood cousins after simultaneous contact with gammexane (hexachlorcyclohexane). Acta med. scand., 161, 447

Johnson, O. (1972) Pesticides '72. Chemical Week, July 26, p. 21

Joslin, E.F., Forney, R.L., Huntington, R.W. & Hayes, W.J., Jr (1958) A fatal case of lindane poisoning. In: Proceedings of the National Association of Coroners, San Diego, California, 1958

Kale, S.C. & Dangwal, S.K. (1971) Hazards during the use of pesticides/insecticides in agricultural farms. In: Proceedings of the Seminar on Pollution and the Human Environment, Bombay, 1970, Bombay, Bhabha Atomic Research Centre, pp. 192-204

Kamada, T. (1971) Hygienic studies on pesticide residues. I. Accumulation of BHC (alpha-, beta-, gamma- and delta-) isomers in rat body and excretion into urine following oral administration. Nippon Eiseigaku Zasshi (Jap. J. Hyg.), 26, 358

Kojima, K. (1972) Epidemiology of organochlorine pesticide pollution. Baioteku (Biotech.), 3, 589

Koransky, W. & Ullberg, S. (1964) Distribution in the brain of ^{14}C-benzenehexachloride: autoradiography study. Biochem. Pharmacol., 13, 1537

Koransky, W., Portig, J. Vohland, H.W. & Klempau, I. (1964) Die Elimination von alpha- und gamma-Hexachlorocyclohexan und ihre Beeinflussung durch Enzyme der Lebermikrosomen. Naunyn-Schmiedebergs Arch. exp. Path. Pharmak., 247, 49

Kroger, M. (1972) Insecticide residues in human milk. J. Pediat., 80, 401

Lichtenberg, J.J., Eichelberger, J.W., Dressman, R.C. & Longbotton, J.E. (1970) Pesticides in surface waters of the United States - a 5-year summary, 1964-1968. Pest. Monit. J., 4, 71

Linder, R.L. & Dahlgren, R.B. (1970) Occurrence of organochlorine insecticides in pheasants of South Dakota. Pest. Monit. J., 3, 227

Loge, J.P. (1965) Aplastic anemia following exposure to benzene hexachloride (lindane). J. amer. med. Ass., 193, 104

Manigold, D.B. & Schulze, J.A. (1969) Pesticides in selected western streams - a progress report. Pest. Monit. J., 3, 124

Martin, R.J. & Duggan, R.E. (1968) Pesticide residues in total diet samples (III). Pest. Monit. J., 1, iv, 11

Martin, W.E. & Nickerson, P.R. (1972) Organochlorine residues in starlings - 1970. Pest. Monit. J., 6, 33

McGill, A.E.J. & Robinson, J. (1968) Organochlorine insecticide residues in complete prepared meals: a 12-month survey in SE England. Fd Cosmet. Toxicol., 6, 45

Morrison, F.O. (1972) A review of the use and place of lindane in the protection of stored products from the ravages of insects pests. Res. Rev., 41, 113

Nagasaki, H., Tomii, S., Mega, T., Marugami, M. & Ito, N. (1971) Development of hepatomas in mice treated with benzene hexachloride. Gann, 62, 431

Nagasaki, H., Tomii, S., Mega, T., Marugami, M. & Ito, N. (1972a) Carcinogenicity of benzene hexachloride (BHC). In: Nakahara, W., Takayama, S., Sugimura, T. & Odashima, S., eds, Topics in Chemical Carcinogenesis, Tokyo, University of Tokyo Press, p. 343

Nagasaki, H., Tomii, S., Mega, T., Marugami, M. & Ito, N. (1972b) Hepatocarcinogenic effect of α-, β-, γ-, and δ-isomers of benzene hexachloride in mice. Gann, 63, 393

Narafu, T. (1971) Pollution of cow's milk and human milk by BHC. Rinsho Eiyo (J. Clin. Nutr.), 39, 26

Orr, J.W. (1948) Absence of carcinogenic activity of benzene hexachloride (Gammexane). Nature (Lond.), 162, 189

Oshiba, K. (1972) Experimental studies on the fate of beta- and gamma-BHC in vivo following daily administration. Osaka Shiritsu Daigaku Igaku Zasshi (J. Osaka City Med. Cent.), 21, 1

Oshiba, K. & Kawakita, H. (1972) Interactions between toxicant and nutrition. V. The fate of β- and γ-BHC in vivo following dietary protein levels. Shokuhin Eiseigaku Zasshi (J. Food Hyg. Soc. Jap.), 13, 383

Radomski, J.L., Deichmann, W.B. & Clizer, E.E. (1968) Pesticide concentrations in the liver, brain and adipose tissue of terminal hospital patients. Fd Cosmet. Toxicol., 6, 209

Saha, J.G. & Sumner, A.K. (1971) Organochlorine insecticide residues in soil from vegetable farms in Saskatchewan. Pest. Monit. J., 5, 28

Schüttmann, U. (1968) Chronische Lebererkrankungen nach beruflicher Einwirkung von Dichlordiphenyltrichloräthan (DDT) und Hexachlor-cyclohexan (HCH). Int. Arch. Gewerbepath. Gewerbehyg., 24, 193

Sieper, H. (1972) Residues et metabolisme. In: Ulmann, E., ed., Lindane, Freiburg i. Br., Verlag K. Schillinger, p. 108

Soós, K., Cieleszky, V. & Tarján, R. (1972) A klórozott szénhidrogének szintjének alakulása a budapesti lakosság zsirszövetében 1970-ben. (The development of the level of chlorinated hydrocarbons in the adipose tissue of the population of Budapest in 1970). Egeszsegtudomany, 16, 70

Spencer, E.Y. (1968) Guide to the Chemicals Used in Crop Protection, 5th ed., Canada Department of Agriculture, Research Branch, No. 1093, p. 304

Stanford Research Institute (1972) Directory of Chemical Producers, Menlo Park, California, p. 773

Stanley, C.W., Barney, J.E., II, Helton, M.R. & Yobs, A.R. (1971) Measurement of atmospheric level of pesticides. Environm. Sci. Technol., 5, 430

Starr, H.G., Jr & Clifford, N.J. (1972) Acute lindane intoxication. Arch. environm. Hlth, 24, 374

Stijve, T. & Cardinale, E. (1972) On the residues associated with the use of technical grade BHC with special reference to the occurrence and determination of three pentachlorocyclohex-1-ene isomers. Mitt. Lebensmitt. Hyg., 63, 142

Szokolay, A., Uhnak, J. & Madaric, A. (1971) Gaschromatographische Bestimmung der Rückstände von chlorierten Insektiziden im Milchfett nach einstufigem Isolations-verfahren. Chem. Zvesti., 25, 453

Tarrant, K.R. & Tatton, J.O'G. (1968) Organochlorine pesticides in rainwater in the British Isles. Nature (Lond.), 219, 725

Tatton, J.O'G. & Ruzicka, J.H.A. (1967) Organochlorine pesticides in Antarctica. Nature (Lond.), 215, 346

Thorpe, E. & Walker, A.I.T. (1973) The toxicology of dieldrin (HEOD). II. Comparative long-term oral toxicity studies in mice with dieldrin, DDT, phenobarbitone, β-BHC and γ-BHC. Fd Cosmet. Toxicol., 11, 433

Tolle, A., Heeschen, W. & Bluethgen, A. (1972) Chlorierte Insektizide, Fasziolizide und Antibiotika in der Milch. Ber. Landwirt., 50, 720

Trautmann, W.L., Chesters, G. & Pionke, H.B. (1968) Organochlorine insecticide composition of randomly selected soils from nine states - 1967. Pest. Monit. J., 2, 93

Trombetti, G. & Gordini, T. (1971) Quantitative determination of the γ-isomer of BHC in technical products and formulations. J. Chromat., 60, 251

Truhaut, R. (1954) Communication au symposium international de la prévention du cancer, Sao Paulo. Cited by FAO/WHO Expert Committee on Pesticide Residues, 1968 Evaluations of some pesticide residues in food. WHO/Food Add. 67.32, p. 130

Tuinstra, L.G.M.Th. (1971) Organochlorine insecticide residues in human milk in the Leiden region. Neth. Milk Dairy J., 25, 24

Uhnak, J. (1971) DDT and other chlorinated insecticides in milk. Vyziva Zdravie, 16, 21

UK Ministry of Agriculture, Fisheries and Food (1973) List of approved products and their uses for farmers and growers, London, pp. 61-63

US Code of Federal Regulations (1972) Washington DC, US Government Printing Office, 29 CFR 1910.93

US Department of Commerce (1970) Chemicals, Business and Defense Services Administration, Washington DC, US Government Printing Office, March 1970, p. 30

US Department of Commerce (1972) Chemicals, Bureau of Domestic Commerce, Washington DC, US Government Printing Office, December 1971/March 1972, pp. 31, 54

US Environmental Protection Agency (1970) EPA Compendium of Registered Pesticides, Washington DC, US Government Printing Office, pp. III-B-6.1 - III-B-6.6

US Environmental Protection Agency (1973) EPA Compendium of Registered Pesticides, Washington DC, US Government Printing Office, pp. III-L-2.1 - III-L-2.12

US Tariff Commission (1946) Synthetic Organic Chemicals, United States Production and Sales, 1945, Washington DC, US Government Printing Office, Second Series, Report No. 157, p. 177

US Tariff Commission (1951) Synthetic Organic Chemicals, United States Production and Sales, 1950, Washington DC, US Government Printing Office, Second Series, Report No. 173, p. 127

US Tariff Commission (1952) Synthetic Organic Chemicals, United States Production and Sales, 1951, Washington DC, US Government Printing Office, Second Series, Report No. 175, p. 54

US Tariff Commission (1964) Synthetic Organic Chemicals, United States Production and Sales, 1963, Washington DC, US Government Printing Office, TC Publication 143, p. 52

US Tariff Commission (1969) Synthetic Organic Chemicals, United States Production and Sales, 1967, Washington DC, US Government Printing Office, TC Publication 295

US Tariff Commission (1973) Imports of Benzenoid Chemicals and Products, 1972, TC Publication 601, August, p. 95

Uporova, G.I. & Shtyler, S.Yu. (1971a) Determination of DDT and hexachlorane in the air by means of thin-layer chromatography. Gig. Tr. Prof. Zabol., 15, 59

Uporova, G.I. & Shtyler, S.Yu. (1971b) Determination of DDT and hexachlorane in food products by thin-layer chromatography. Gig. Sanit., 36, 97

Uyeta, M., Taue, S., Chikazawa, K. & Nishimoto, T. (1971) Pesticides translocated in food - organochlorine pesticides in the total diet. Shokuhin Eiseigaku Zasshi (J. Fd Hyg. Soc. Jap.), 12, 445

Wakimoto, T., Tatsukawa, R. & Ogawa, T. (1970) Air pollution by pesticides. II. Air pollution by BHC. Taiki Osen Kenkyu, 5, 92

Walker, C.H., Hamilton, G.A. & Harrison, R.B. (1967) Organochlorine insecticide residues in wild birds in Britain. J. Sci. Fd Agric., 18, 123

Ware, G.W. & Naber, E.C. (1961) Lindane in eggs and chicken tissues. J. econ. Entomol., 54, 675

Wassermann, M., Iliescu, S., Mandric, G. & Horvath, P. (1960) Toxic hazards during DDT- and BHC-spraying of forests against Lymantria monacha. Arch. industr. Hlth, 21, 503

West, I. (1967) Lindane and hematologic reactions. Arch. environm. Hlth, 15, 97

Wheatley, G.A. & Hardman, J.A. (1965) Indications of the presence of organochlorine insecticides in rainwater in central England. Nature (Lond.), 207, 486

WHO (1972) 1971 Evaluations of some pesticide residues in food. WHO Pesticide Residues Series, No. 1, pp. 315, 338, 340

Wiersma, G.B., Taï, H. & Sand, P.F. (1972) Pesticide residue levels in soils, FY 1969 - National Soils Monitoring Program. Pest. Monit. J., 6, 194

Williams, S. & Mills, P.A. (1964) Residues in milk of cows fed rations containing low concentrations of five chlorinated hydrocarbon pesticides. J. Ass. off. analyt. Chem., 47, 1124

Woodliff, H.J., Connor, P.M. & Scopa, J. (1966) Aplastic anemia associated with insecticides. Med. J. Austral., 1, 628

CHLOROBENZILATE

Chlorobenzilate is the common name recommended by the International Standards Organization (except in the United States) for ethyl 4,4'-dichlorobenzilate. Two reviews on this compound are available (FAO/WHO, 1969, 1973a).

1. Chemical and Physical Data

1.1 Synonyms and trade names

Chem. Abstr. No.: 510-15-6

Akar; Benzilan; Chlorobenzilat; 4,4'-dichlorobenzilic acid ethyl ester; ethyl p,p'-dichlorobenzilate; ethyl 4,4'-dichlorobenzilate; ethyl 4,4'-dichlorodiphenyl glycollate; ethyl 4,4'-dichlorophenyl glycollate; ethyl 2-hydroxy-2,2-bis(4-chlorophenyl)acetate; ethyl ester of 4,4'-dichlorobenzilic acid; Folbex; G-23992; Geigy 338; Kop-Mite

1.2 Chemical formula and molecular weight

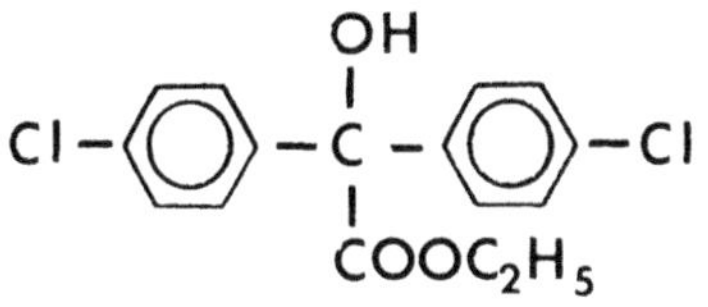

$Cl-\bigcirc-\underset{\underset{COOC_2H_5}{|}}{\overset{\overset{OH}{|}}{C}}-\bigcirc-Cl$ $C_{16}H_{14}Cl_2O_3$ Mol. wt: 325.2

1.3 Chemical and physical properties of the pure substance

(a) *Description*: Yellow solid (Martin, 1971). Yellowish, viscous liquid (Bartsch et al., 1971)

(b) *Melting-point*: 35-37°C

(c) *Boiling-point*: 141-142°C at 0.06 mm Hg

(d) *Solubility*: Insoluble in water; soluble in most organic solvents and petroleum oils

(e) *Volatility*: Vapour pressure is 2.2×10^{-6} mm Hg at 20°C

(f) *Chemical reactivity*: Hydrolyzed by alkalis and strong acids

1.4 Technical products and impurities

The technical product, with a specific gravity of D_4^{20} = 1.2816 and a refractive index of n_D^{20} = 1.5727, is a brownish liquid which contains about 93% of the chemical.

Chlorobenzilate is commercially available in the United States as a technical grade having a minimum content of 90% active ingredient (the chemical nature of the impurities is not known). It is also offered for sale as a 45.5% active emulsifiable concentrate or a 25% active wettable powder and can be formulated as dusts and aerosol products.

2. Production, Use, Occurrence and Analysis

2.1 Production and use[1]

It is not known when chlorobenzilate was first synthesized, but it was first introduced for use as an acaricide in 1952. It is made by the reaction of dichlorobenzilic acid with ethyl sulphate (Martin, 1971).

Only one company in the US manufactures chlorobenzilate, and it has been estimated that one million kg were produced in 1971 (Johnson, 1972).

It is believed that one company in Switzerland makes chlorobenzilate; and Berg (1971) has indicated that it is produced in Israel.

The only known use for chlorobenzilate is as an acaricide, although Merck & Co. (1968) list it as a synergist for DDT. As of May 31, 1969 chlorobenzilate was approved in the US for use on 11 crops (mostly fruits and nuts), and tolerances for residues in several raw agricultural commodities were in effect (US Environmental Protection Agency, 1969).

In 1972, total usage of chlorobenzilate in California, a major agricultural state, amounted to 29 thousand kg. Almost half of this was used on almonds, and nearly one-third on cotton (California Department of Agriculture, 1973). Chlorobenzilate has been used as a pre-harvest contact acaricide in many countries.

---

[1] Data from Chemical Information Services, Stanford Research Institute, USA

An indication of the uses of chlorobenzilate can be derived from the FAO/WHO recommended tolerances and practical limits for this substance on the following food products: apples, pears, citrus fruits, grapes, melons, almonds, walnuts (shelled), tomatoes and whole milk (FAO/WHO, 1973b).

2.2 Occurrence

Controlled feeding studies in sheep and cattle showed that residues of chlorobenzilate were found in fat of cattle only at the highest feeding level (340 mg/animal/day) (FAO/WHO, 1969).

Roth (1958) found 0.2-1.5 ppm in pears. The concentration in apples after one application of a 62 g/100 ml solution of chlorobenzilate was 4.98 ppm one day after treatment; this decreased over 8 days to 4.33 ppm and after 39 days to 0.9 ppm (FAO/WHO, 1969). In apples and citrus fruits chlorobenzilate was found exclusively in the peel, from which it disappeared slowly (Gunther et al., 1955).

Corneliussen (1972) found no intake from food in the US. No data are available on residues in air and water.

The acceptable daily intake for man has been established at 0-0.02 mg/kg bw/day (FAO/WHO, 1969).

2.3 Analysis

A general approach to the analysis of organochlorine pesticides has been given in the preamble (p. 16).

A review on chlorobenzilate, including its analytical determination, is given by Bartsch et al. (1971).

A spectrophotometric method for determinations on citrus fruits is described by Blinn et al. (1954). The method was tested and modified for different types of crops by Harris (1955), by Baker & Skerret (1958) and by Margot & Stammbach (1964). A gas chromatographic method, for analyses of grapes and cotton seed, is described by Beckmann & Benevue (1964).

3. Biological Data Relevant to the Evaluation of Carcinogenic Risk to Man

3.1 Carcinogenicity and related studies in animals

(a) Oral administration

Mouse: In a study published as a preliminary note, 18 male and 18 female (C57BL/6 x C3H/Anf)Fl mice and similar numbers of (C57BL/6 x AKR)Fl mice were given single doses of 215 mg/kg bw chlorobenzilate by stomach tube when the animals were 7 days of age; the same absolute amount was given daily until the animals were 4 weeks of age, when they were administered a diet containing 603 ppm chlorobenzilate. The experiment lasted 83 weeks. Hepatomas were found in both strains, but only in males, the incidence being 9/17 in (C57BL/6 x C3H/Anf)Fl mice compared with 8/79 in male controls and 7/17 in (C57BL/6 x AKR)Fl mice compared with 5/90 in male controls. Incidences of other tumours were similar in treated and control animals (Innes et al., 1969).

Rat: In a small study, groups of 20 CF rats of each sex were fed a diet containing either 0, 50 (males only) or 500 ppm technical chlorobenzilate for 2 years. Some 13-14 rats/treatment group and 12-16 male and female controls were alive at the end of the experiment. Tumours occurred sporadically in treated and control animals (Horn et al., 1955).

In a study which has not been published in detail, 4 groups of 30 rats of each sex were fed a diet containing either 0, 40, 125 or 400 ppm of the active ingredient as a 25% wettable formulation. Treatment lasted 2 years. Lifespan results are not reported, but incidences of neoplasms are reported to be unrelated to the administration of the compound (cited in FAO/WHO, 1969; Bartsch et al., 1971). (The Working Group was unable to evaluate the information given in this study due to inadequate reporting.)

3.2 Other relevant biological data

(a) Metabolism and storage in animals

When daily doses of 12.8 mg/kg bw chlorobenzilate were given orally to male mongrel dogs on 5 days a week for 35 weeks, 42.67% of the total dose was excreted in the urine; in a female receiving the same dose, 41.84% was excreted unchanged in the urine. When higher doses of 64.1 mg/kg bw/day were given, the corresponding values were 21.77% and 15.13%, respectively. At termination of the study the compound could not be detected in blood, liver, kidney, fat, muscle or brain (Horn et al., 1955).

Rat liver homogenate metabolizes chlorobenzilate in vitro, and p-chlorobenzoic acid was identified as an end product (Knowles & Ahmad, 1971).

3.3 Observations in man

No data were available to the Working Group.

4. Comments on Data Reported and Evaluation[1]

4.1 Animal data

Chlorobenzilate was tested in a preliminary study by the oral route in two strains of mice and produced an increased incidence of hepatomas in males of both strains.

Reports of feeding studies in rats were considered inadequate for evaluation.

4.2 Human data

No epidemiological studies were available to the Working Group.

---

[1] See also the section "Animal Data in Relation to the Evaluation of Risk to Man" in the introduction to this volume.

5. References

Baker, E.A. & Skerrett, E.J. (1958) Determination of DDT and chlorobenzilate occurring together in spray deposits. Analyst, 83, 447

Bartsch, E., Eberle, D., Ramsreiner, K., Tomann, A. & Spindler, M. (1971) The carbinole acaricides: chlorobenzilate and chloropropylate. Res. Rev., 39, 1

Beckman, H. & Bevenue, A. (1964) Microcoulometric gas chromatographic analysis of grapes and cottonseed for chlorobenzilate residues. J. agric. Fd Chem., 12, 183

Berg, G.L., ed. (1971) Farm Chemicals Handbook, Willoughby, Ohio, Meister, p. D127

Blinn, R.C., Gunther, F.A. & Kolbezen, M.J. (1954) Microdetermination of the acaricide p,p'-dichlorobenzilate (chlorobenzilate). J. agric. Fd Chem., 2, 1080

California Department of Agriculture (1973) Pesticide Use Report, 1972, Sacramento, pp. 42-43

Corneliussen, P.E. (1972) Pesticide residues in total diet samples (VI). Pest. Monit. J., 5, 313

FAO/WHO (1969) 1968 Evaluations of some pesticide residues in food. FAO/PL/1968/M/9/1; WHO/Food Add./69.35, p. 45

FAO/WHO (1973a) 1972 Evaluations of some pesticide residues in food. WHO Pesticide Residues Series, No. 2 (in press)

FAO/WHO (1973b) Pesticide residues in food. Report of the 1972 Joint FAO/WHO Meeting. Wld Hlth Org. techn. Rep. Ser., No. 525

Gunther, F.A., Jeppson, L.R. & Wacker, G.E. (1955) Persistence of chlorobenzilate residues in mature lemon fruits. J. econ. Entomol., 48, 372

Harris, H.J. (1955) Colorimetric determination of ethyl 4,4'-dichlorobenzilate (chlorobenzilate) as a spray residue. J. agric. Fd Chem., 3, 939

Horn, H.J., Bruce, R.B. & Paynter, O.E. (1955) Toxicology of chlorobenzilate. J. agric. Fd Chem., 3, 752

Innes, J.R.M., Ulland, B.M., Valerio, M.G., Petrucelli, L., Fishbein, L., Hart, E.R., Pallotta, A.J., Bates, R.R., Falk, H.L., Gart, J.J., Klein, M., Mitchell, I. & Peters, J. (1969) Bioassay of pesticides and industrial chemicals for tumorigenicity in mice. A preliminary note. J. nat. Cancer Inst., 42, 1101

Johnson, O. (1972) Pesticides '72. Chemical Week, June 21, p. 48

Knowles, C.O. & Ahmad, S. (1971) Comparative metabolism of chlorobenzilate, chloropropylate and bromopropylate acaricides by rat hepatic enzymes. Canad. J. Physiol. Pharmacol., 49, 590

Margot, A. & Stammbach, K. (1964) Chlorobenzilate. In: Zweig, G., ed., Analytic Methods for Pesticides, Plant Regulators and Food Additives, Vol. 2, London, New York, Academic Press, p. 65

Martin, H., ed. (1971) Pesticide Manual. Basic Information on the Chemicals used as Active Components of Pesticides. 2nd ed., Ombersley, British Crop Protection Council, p. 97

Merck & Co. (1968) The Merck Index, Rahway, N.J., p. 240

Roth, F.J. (1958) A one-shot, two-filter application of the Schechter method for mixed DDT and chlorobenzilate spray residues. J. Ass. off. analyt. Chem., 41, 662

US Environmental Protection Agency (1969) EPA Compendium of Registered Pesticides, Washington DC, US Government Printing Office, p. III-E-6

DDT AND ASSOCIATED SUBSTANCES

DDT is the common name approved by the International Standards Organization for the technical product of which 1,1,1-trichloro-2,2-di-(4-chlorophenyl)ethane (p,p'-DDT) is the predominant component. Several reviews on this compound are available (FAO/WHO, 1967, 1968, 1969, 1970).

1. Chemical and Physical Data

1.1 Synonyms and trade names

(a) <u>DDT</u>

Chem. Abstr. No.: MX 8017343

Arkotine; Dicophane; Estonate; Gesarol; Guesarol; Neocid; technical chlorophenothane; Zerdane

(b) <u>p,p'-DDT</u>

Chem. Abstr. No.: 50-29-3

α,α-Bis(p-chlorophenyl) β,β,β-trichlorethane; 2,2-bis(p-chlorophenyl)-1,1,1-trichloroethane; chlorophenothane; p,p'-dichlorodiphenyltrichloroethane; 4,4'-dichlorodiphenyltrichloroethane; trichlorobis(4'-chlorophenyl)ethane; 1,1,1-trichloro-2,2-bis(p-chlorophenyl)ethane

(c) <u>o,p'-DDT</u>

Chem. Abstr. No.: 789-02-6

o,p'-Dichlorodiphenyltrichloroethane; 1,1,1-trichloro-2-(o-chlorophenyl)-2-(p-chlorophenyl)ethane; β,β,β-trichloro-α-(o-chlorophenyl)-α-(p-chlorophenyl)ethane

(d) <u>p,p'-TDE (DDD)</u>*

Chem. Abstr. No.: 72-54-8

---

* Although the abbreviation DDD is incorrect, it is still commonly used in papers relating to the biological effects of TDE.

1,1-Dichloro-2,2'-bis(p-chlorophenyl)ethane; dichlorodiphenyl-dichloroethane; p,p'-DDD; Rothane

(e) <u>p,p'-DDE</u>

Chem. Abstr. No.: 72-55-9

1,1-Dichloro-2,2-bis(p-chlorophenyl)ethylene

1.2 Chemical formulae and molecular weights

<u>p,p'-DDT</u>

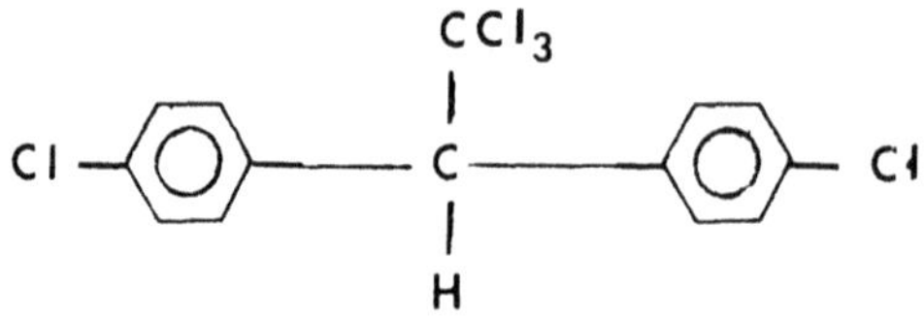

Cl–⟨⟩–C(CCl$_3$)(H)–⟨⟩–Cl $C_{14}H_9Cl_5$

Mol. wt: 354.5

<u>o,p'-DDT</u>

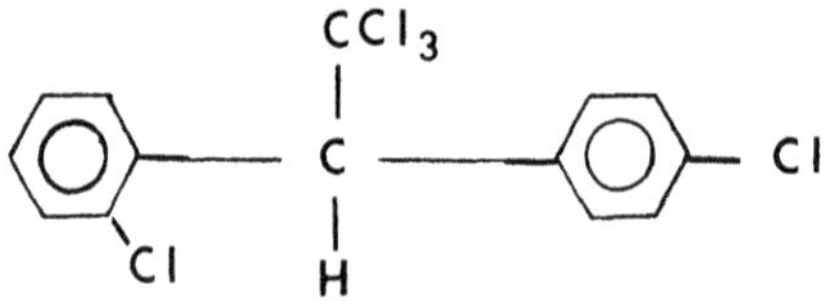

⟨⟩(Cl)–C(CCl$_3$)(H)–⟨⟩–Cl $C_{14}H_9Cl_5$

Mol. wt: 354.5

<u>p,p'-TDE (DDD)</u>

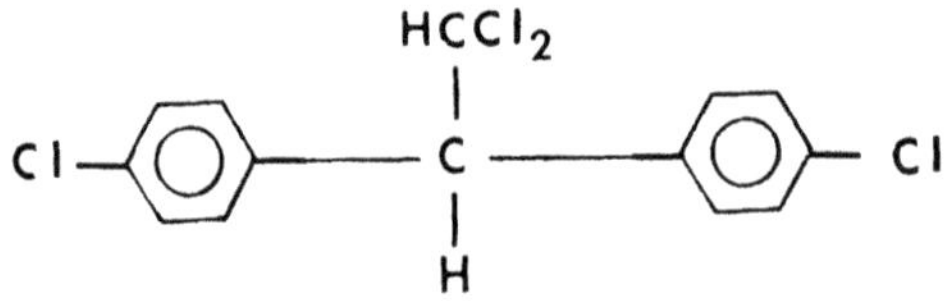

Cl–⟨⟩–C(HCCl$_2$)(H)–⟨⟩–Cl $C_{14}H_{10}Cl_4$

Mol. wt: 320.0

<u>p,p'-DDE</u>

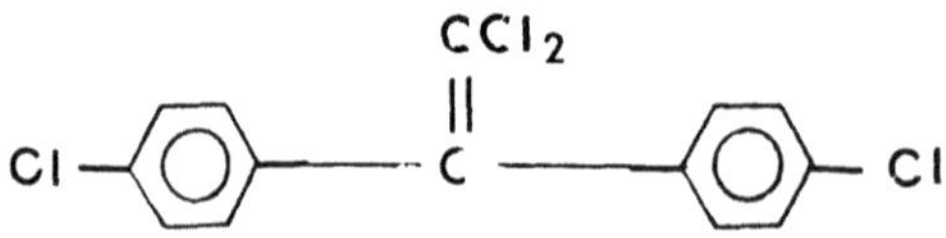

Cl–⟨⟩–C(=CCl$_2$)–⟨⟩–Cl $C_{14}H_{10}Cl_4$

Mol. wt: 318.0

1.3 Chemical and physical properties of the pure substance

<u>p,p'-DDT</u>

(<u>a</u>) <u>Description</u>:   Colourless crystals

(<u>b</u>) <u>Melting-point</u>:   108.5°C

(c) Solubility: Practically insoluble in water and very soluble in fats and most organic solvents

(d) Volatility: Vapour pressure is 1.9×10^{-7} mm Hg at $20°C$

(e) Chemical reactivity: DDT dehydrochlorinates at temperatures above its melting-point to yield DDE; the reaction is catalyzed by ferric and aluminium chloride and by UV light. It dehydrochlorinates in organic solvents in the presence of alkalis or organic bases, is stable to strong acids and can withstand acid permanganate oxidation (Martin, 1971).

o,p'-DDT

(a) Description: White, crystalline solid

(b) Melting-point: 74-75°C (74.2°C)

(c) Solubility: Water, 0.085 mg/l at 25°C; soluble in fat and most organic solvents

(d) Chemical reactivity: Stable to concentrated sulphuric acid

p,p'-TDE (DDD)

(a) Description: Colourless crystals

(b) Melting-point: 109-110°C

(c) Solubility: Similar to that of p,p'-DDT

(d) Chemical reactivity: Similar to that of p,p'-DDT, but it is more slowly hydrolyzed by alkalis

p,p'-DDE

(a) Description: White, crystalline solid

(b) Melting-point: 88-89°C (88.4°C)

(c) Solubility: Water, 0.12 mg/l at 25°C; soluble in fat and most organic solvents

(d) Chemical reactivity: Stable to concentrated sulphuric acid. It may be oxidized to p,p'-dichlorobenzophenone, a reaction catalyzed by UV radiation (Metcalf, 1966)

1.4 Technical products and impurities

(a) DDT

The technical product is a waxy solid of indefinite m.p. and of similar solubility to p,p'-DDT.

Technical DDT is a mixture of isomers containing some 65-80% of p,p'-DDT and up to 14 other components. The major impurities are: o,p'-DDT (15-21%); p,p'-TDE (up to 4%); 1-(p-chlorophenyl)-2,2,2-trichloroethanol (up to 1.5%); traces of o,o'-DDT; and traces of bis (p-chlorophenyl)sulphone (Metcalf, 1966). Up to 1% m,p'-DDT may be present in some technical DDT (Tomatis et al., 1972).

Prior to 1973, DDT was available in the United States in the following grades and forms: (1) technical (used in chip or flake form by pesticide formulators); (2) purified; (3) aerosol; and (4) U.S.P. as chlorophenothane (5-10% DDT) - a powder used medicinally as a lotion, emulsion, ointment or powder.

(b) TDE (DDD)

TDE is available as a technical grade product containing mostly p,p'-TDE, with a setting-point not less than 86°C. It contains related compounds as impurities (the major one being up to 10% of the o,p'-isomer). TDE is also formulated into wettable powders, emulsifiable concentrates and dusts (Martin, 1971).

2. Production, Use, Occurrence and Analysis

Several comprehensive review articles on pesticides (including DDT) have been written recently (Faust, 1972; Lawless et al., 1972; Metcalf, 1966; US Department of Health, Education & Welfare, 1969).

2.1 Production and use[1]

(a) DDT

Technical DDT is made by condensing chloral hydrate with chlorobenzene

---

[1] Data from Chemical Information Services, Stanford Research Institute, USA

in the presence of sulphuric acid. It was first synthesized in 1874, but it was not until 1939 that Müller and his coworkers (Läuger et al., 1944) discovered its insecticidal properties. By 1943, low-cost production methods had been developed, and commercial production had begun. Production of DDT continued to increase until 1969 when the US Department of Agriculture announced that DDT could no longer be used in the US unless its use was justified by documentation. In June 1972, the Environmental Protection Agency issued a ban (effective December 31, 1972) on all but minor uses of DDT (an appeal is pending).

US production of DDT in 1971 has been estimated to have been 20 million kg (Lawless et al., 1972). This represented a sharp decline from the 82 million kg produced in 1963 (US Tariff Commission, 1964) and from the 56 million kg produced in 1969 (US Tariff Commission, 1971). At the present time there is only one US producer, with a plant capacity of 39 million kg per year (Anon., 1972a).

US imports of DDT amounted to 200 thousand kg in 1972 (US Tariff Commission, 1973), and exports of DDT and DDT-containing products totalled 16 million kg. These exports included: 12 million kg of technical DDT (countries receiving over 450 thousand kg were Guatemala, Nicaragua, Brazil, India, Australia and the Republic of South Africa); 2.3 million kg of DDT preparations (excluding household and industrial) containing less than 75% DDT; and 1.4 million kg of DDT preparations (excluding household and industrial) containing 75% or more DDT (US Bureau of the Census, 1973).

Producers of technical DDT in Europe in 1972 or 1973 were as follows (the number of producers is given in parentheses): France (3), Italy (5), Spain (10) and the United Kingdom (1) (Chemical Information Services Ltd., 1973; Economic Documentation Office, 1973; Ragno, 1972). However, as of 1972, there were reportedly only three major producers left in Europe and North America (Anon., 1972b). DDT is also known to be produced in: Brazil, where production was 3 million kg in 1969 and is believed to be increasing (US Department of Commerce, 1972); Israel, where the total capacity in 1970 was 350 thousand kg (US Department of Commerce, 1970);

and India, where production for 1971-72 was 4 million kg and was expected to increase (Anon., 1972c). Japan produced 4.6 million kg in 1970 (Hayashi, 1971).

In 1966 it was estimated that 38% of all DDT used in the US was for agricultural purposes, 12% for residential uses, 25% for institutional markets and 25% for exports (Metcalf, 1966). DDT has been used for the control of hundreds of insect pests in orchards, gardens, fields and forests. It has also been used widely in public health measures, e.g., as a mosquito larvicide, as a residual spray for the eradication of malaria in dwellings and as a dust in mass human delousing programmes for typhus control. In addition, DDT has been used for mothproofing, where fabrics are impregnated with 0.25-0.75% DDT or sprayed with a 0.5% DDT solution (Metcalf, 1966).

By 1972, only 4.5-6.4 million kg of DDT were expected to be consumed in the US (Anon., 1972d; Lawless et al., 1972). Use on cotton crops has been estimated to have accounted for 67-90% of the total US consumption in 1972, and the remaining DDT was used primarily on peanut and soybean crops. US consumption of DDT in 1973 has been limited to use in public health measures and for three minor uses - treatments of green peppers, onions and sweet potatoes in storage (Anon., 1972e; Schorr, 1972).

The US Environmental Protection Agency (1973) has proposed a list of toxic pollutants, which includes DDT, DDE and TDE. If this list is adopted, effluent standards restricting or prohibiting discharges of these chemicals into streams may come into effect.

On a worldwide basis, DDT is consumed primarily in the prevention of malaria, yellow fever and sleeping sickness and as such is distributed by the World Health Organization. Approximately 50% of world production in 1971 was used in this way (Anon., 1972a).

Quantities of DDT and related compounds used in or sold for agricultural purposes in 1970 were as follows (thousand kg): Austria (20.5); Botswana (2.0); Canada (287.0); Ceylon (16.6); Colombia (980.0); Czechoslovakia (270.0); Egypt (3,457.0); El Salvador (466.0); Federal Republic of Germany (152.0); Finland (6.1); Ghana (0.3); Guatemala

(380.0); Hungary (20.6); Iceland (0.3); Israel (10.0); Italy (2,178.0); Japan (401.0); Khmer (46.8); Kuwait (0.2); Madagascar (176.0); Ryukyu Islands (0.3); Sudan (269.0); Upper Volta (1.5); Uruguay (5.0) (FAO, 1972).

An indication of some uses for DDT can be derived from the FAO/WHO recommended tolerances and practical limits on DDT, TDE and DDE, singly, or in combinations. Included are residue limit values for apples, pears, peaches, apricots, plums, citrus and tropical fruits, cherries, strawberries, vegetables (root vegetables and others), nuts, milk and milk products and eggs (FAO/WHO, 1973).

In the Federal Republic of Germany, DDT will be permitted for use in some forestry applications until the end of 1974 (BBLF, 1972); in Japan, its use on crops is prohibited (Anon., 1972f); and in Portugal, since 1970, DDT has been restricted to uses other than on human and animal foods (Chaby Nunes & Oliveira Nobre, 1972). DDT is used only for control of pine-weevils on conifers in Norway (Stenersen, 1972), and its application is not permitted at all in Switzerland (EFOWG; EFLP; SFRA, 1972). In the UK, the use of DDT alone or in combination with other pesticides is permitted, with a number of limitations (UK Ministry of Agriculture, Fisheries and Food, 1973). In 1971, the USSR issued tolerances for residues in vegetables, fruit (except strawberries and raspberries) and forage intended for animal consumption (Melnikov & Schevchenko, 1971).

(b) TDE (DDD)

The insecticidal properties of technical TDE were first described in 1944, and it was introduced commercially in the US in 1945. Chlorination of ethanol gives a chlorinated mixture which is then condensed with chloral, resulting in a product containing 90% p,p'-TDE and some o,p'-TDE (Martin, 1971).

Two companies in the US produce TDE. No estimates of the quantity produced were found in the trade literature; it is believed to be quite small at present, although it may have amounted to several million kilograms in earlier years.

TDE reportedly has proved less effective against moths than DDT, but it is superior against some other insects (e.g., tomato hornworms) (Metcalf, 1966).

The pure o,p'-TDE isomer, specially synthesized, has been used in the treatment of adrenocortical carcinoma (Bergenstal et al., 1960) and in the treatment of the overproduction of adrenal cortical steroids (Bledsoe et al., 1964; Gallagher et al., 1962; Southern et al., 1966a,b; Verdon et al., 1962; Wallace et al., 1961).

The US Environmental Protection Agency (1973) has proposed a list of toxic pollutants, which includes TDE, DDT and DDE. If this list is adopted, effluent standards restricting or prohibiting discharges of these chemicals into streams may come into effect.

The use of TDE was prohibited in Switzerland in 1972 (Anon., 1972g), and the USSR has established tolerance levels for TDE in grain, vegetables and fruit (Melnikov & Schevchenko, 1971).

2.2 Occurrence

(a) Occupational exposure

Several studies have been carried out of the exposure of workers manufacturing and formulating DDT and of those applying it. Indications of exposure have been determined either by direct or indirect measurements of DDT levels in blood (Edmundson et al., 1969) and body fat (Hayes et al., 1956) and by determination of DDA levels in urine (Durham et al., 1965; Ortelee, 1958). Using direct methods of measurement, estimations of potential dermal exposure ranged from 84 mg/hr for outdoor spraying (Hayes, 1959) to 1,755 mg/hr for indoor spraying (Wolfe et al., 1959, 1967). Values of 212 mg/hr were found during forest spraying (Wassermann et al., 1960) and of 524.5 mg/hr for formulating plant workers (Wolfe & Armstrong, 1971).

Estimation of potential respiratory exposure ranged from 0.11 mg/hr for outdoor spraying to 7.1 mg/hr for indoor spraying (Wolfe et al., 1959), with values of 4.92 mg/hr for forest spraying (Wassermann et al., 1960) and of 14.1 mg/hr for formulating plant workers (Wolfe & Armstrong, 1971).

Laws et al. (1967) estimated that the average daily intake of DDT by 20 men with high occupational exposure was 17.5-18 mg/man/day as compared with an average of 0.04 mg/man/day for the general population; determinations were made indirectly from levels of DDT stored in fat and excretion of DDA in urine.

(b) Air and rain

The occurrence of DDT in air has been reviewed by Finkelstein (1969); the concentration was found to vary according to the locality and the season. In general, the concentration was lower in urban than in agricultural areas, with higher levels being found during the summer: the highest levels were found when pesticide spraying was reported. There was no apparent correlation of level with rainfall, but after several days of rain the level usually decreased (Finkelstein, 1969; Stanley et al., 1971). Concentrations of DDT ranged from 0.1 ng/m^3 (lower limit of detection) to as high as 1.56 µg/m^3 in nine localities of various parts of the US (Stanley et al., 1971), and in London and suburbs very small quantities (10 g "DDT"/10^{12}g of air) were detected (Abbott et al., 1966). Antommaria et al. (1965) found up to 1.14 µg p,p'-DDT/m^3 of air in Pittsburgh; in airborne dust, levels of 0.6 mg/kg DDT and 0.2 mg/kg DDE (Cohen & Pinkerton, 1966), 2.7-88 µg/kg p,p'-DDT (Risebrough et al., 1968) and averages of 108 and 57 x 10^{-15} g/m^3 p,p'-DDT and 27 and 9 x 10^{-15} g/m^3 p,p'-DDE (Prospero & Seba, 1972; Seba & Prospero, 1971) have been found. In agricultural communities, 0.1-22 ng DDT/m^3 were detected, and during pesticide applications the concentration ranged from 100-8000 ng/m^3 (Tabor, 1966). Tabor (1965) has thus calculated a possible daily respiratory intake of 0.2 to 0.8 µg DDT/24 hrs.

The average concentration found in rainwater ranged from 3 ng p,p'-DDT/l (Bevenue et al., 1972; Wheatley & Hardman, 1965) to 187 ng/l DDT (Cohen & Pinkerton, 1966). Levels of 40 ng o,p'- + p,p'-DDT/kg have been found in Antarctic snow (Peterle, 1969).

(c) Soil and water

Soil concentrations of DDT vary according to the land use, and many studies of the DDT content of agricultural soil have been carried out

(Deubert & Zuckerman, 1969; Saha & Sumner, 1971; Sand et al., 1972; Seal et al., 1967; Wiersma et al., 1972a). In general, orchard and vegetable-growing areas showed higher DDT contamination than did corn- and hay-growing areas (Trautmann et al., 1968). Average DDT concentrations (o,p'- + p,p'-DDT + DDE) ranged from 0.5 ppm for "soybean soil" (McCaskill et al., 1970) to as much as 10.1 ppm for "orchard soil" (Stenersen & Friestad, 1969). Average total DDT concentrations (DDT + DDE + TDE) ranged from 0.85 ppm for "alfalfa soil" (Ware et al., 1968) to 15.10 ppm for onion-growing soil (Wiersma et al., 1972b). In a review of published data Woodwell et al. (1971) estimate that agricultural soils in the US contain an average content of "DDT" approaching 0.168 g/m^2.

Edwards (1966) has estimated that the average time for 95% disappearance of DDT would be 10 years (range, 4-30 years) with an average of about 50% (26-78%) remaining after three years. However, Chisholm & McPhee (1972) have estimated that more than 50% of applied DDT would remain in soils for at least 15 years.

DDT has been found in most surface waters that have been investigated, in drinking-water at various locations and in ocean marine life. For a review of DDT concentrations in water, see Faust (1972). In drinking-water, an average of 1 ng p,p'-DDT/l has been found (Bevenue et al., 1972); and Wolter (1972) detected 0.06 mg DDT/l in water used for drinking 17 days after aerial spraying of DDT.

Many studies have been carried out of the occurrence of DDT, DDE and TDE in surface waters, mostly in rivers and lakes in the US. Concentrations found ranged from 0-0.8 µg/l (Brown & Nishioka, 1967; Herzel, 1972; Johnson & Morris, 1971; Lichtenberg et al., 1970; Manigold & Schulze, 1969). After aerial spraying the DDT content of surface waters varied from <0.001-0.004 mg/l (Wolter & Rugenstein, 1971).

(d) <u>Animals and plants</u>

DDT is stored in tissues, in particular in adipose tissue, and in liver, brain and muscle of mammals, fish, reptiles and birds; it is also stored in insects, algae, plankton and in the eggs of fish and birds.

Fish can build up mg/kg concentrations of DDT from ng/l levels in water (Reinert, 1970); a review of the ratios of DDT concentrations in algae and fish to those in water is given by Bevenue et al. (1972) - they were found to range from 800:1 to 20,000:1.

Many determinations of DDT concentration in fish (including shellfish) from rivers, lakes, estuaries and the sea have been reported (Bradshaw et al., 1972; Burnett, 1971; Earnest & Benville, 1971; Henderson et al., 1971; Stenersen, 1972). The highest concentrations, up to 187.5 ppm DDT, were found in fatty tissue (Johnson & Lew, 1970).

DDT has also been detected in many bird species (domestic and wild) at concentrations ranging from <0.001-126 ppm DDT in fat, 0.02-19.2 ppm in liver, 0.03-1.06 ppm in muscle and 0.3-4.5 ppm in eggs (Baetcke et al., 1972). Average concentrations in eagle eggs ranged from traces to 21.3 ppm DDT (Wiemeyer et al., 1972). Many other wild animals have been examined for their DDT content, e.g., reptiles (Culley & Applegate, 1967), frogs (Cory et al., 1970), sea lions (Le Boeuf & Bonnell, 1971), seals (Anas & Wilson, 1970) and whales (Wolman & Wilson, 1970).

(e) Food

In the US, the UK and Japan a series of analyses of total diets have been carried out (Abbott et al., 1969; Corneliussen, 1969, 1970, 1972; Cummings, 1966; Duggan & Corneliussen, 1972; Duggan & Lipscomb, 1969; Duggan & Weatherwax, 1967; Duggan et al., 1966, 1967, 1971; Egan et al., 1966; Martin & Duggan, 1968; McGill & Robinson, 1968; Robinson & McGill, 1966; Uyeta et al., 1971). As a consequence of restrictive legislation approved recently in many countries, the DDT content of food is generally decreasing, and a clear decline in the levels of DDT and its analogues has been found (Duggan & Corneliussen, 1972).

In meat, fish and poultry the concentration of total DDT (DDT + DDE + TDE) has decreased from a maximum value of 3.2 ppm in 1967 (Duggan et al., 1967) to a maximum value of 0.9 ppm in 1972 (Corneliussen, 1972). In beef and pork fat samples, Adamczyk (1971) detected more than 7 ppm DDT + DDE, but in none of the liver or meat samples did the content exceed 1 ppm.

A Joint FAO/WHO meeting in 1968 (FAO/WHO, 1969) summarized the data on controlled uses of DDT on and around poultry. Feeding levels of 0.05-0.45 ppm for 13 weeks resulted in residues of 0.06 ppm p,p'-DDT + 0.03 ppm DDE to 0.28 ppm p,p'-DDT + 0.09 ppm DDE in the whole eggs (94% in the yolk, 6% in the white) (Cummings et al., 1966). Wright et al. (1972) analyzed the egg yolks of chickens given daily doses of 10 mg/kg bw p,p'-DDT orally: after 60 days, residues were approximately 260 ppm p,p'-DDT + 70 ppm DDE.

Dairy products acquire DDT either through feeding or spraying of the animals and their dwellings. The probable residue level of DDT and its metabolites in milk is about 3.8% of the residue content of the feed (Saha, 1969). In many European countries and in the US, the DDT levels in dairy products have decreased since 1965; average values for total DDT ranged in different countries from 0.008-0.4 ppm on a fat basis (Bjerk & Sakshaug, 1969 (butter); Duggan, 1967 (milk); Frank et al., 1970 (milk); McGill & Robinson, 1968 (milk); Tolle et al., 1972 (milk, butter and cheese); Uhnak, 1971 (butter)). In Denmark, the concentration in milk fat declined from 0.15 ppm DDT + DDE in 1964 to 0.12 ppm in 1965 and 0.08 ppm in 1966, and in butter from 0.08 ppm in 1964 to 0.07 ppm in 1965 and to 0.06 ppm in 1966 (Bro-Rasmussen et al., 1968).

In the US, the concentration of total DDT in dairy products found in total diet studies decreased from a maximum value of 0.8 ppm in 1967 (Duggan et al., 1967) to 0.3 ppm in 1972 (Corneliussen, 1972). Practical residue limits for milk have been set at 0.05 ppm and for milk products at 1.25 ppm (FAO/WHO, 1969).

Average concentrations of p,p'-DDT found in human milk range from 0.05-0.2 ppm (Egan et al., 1965; Heyndrickx & Maes, 1969; Laug et al., 1951; Quinby et al., 1965); higher levels of total DDT (up to 0.6 ppm) were found by Hagyard et al. (1973), and 2.4 ppm (Kroger, 1972) and 8.2 ppm (Engst & Knoll, 1971) have been found in human milk fat.

Many analyses have been made of DDT residues in fruits and vegetables. In vegetables, the maximum value of DDT + DDE + TDE ranged from about 0.05 ppm (Corneliussen, 1972) to 0.2 ppm (Corneliussen, 1969), the highest amounts being found in leafy vegetables (spinach, broccoli, etc.) and in legumes (peas, beans, etc.) (0.3 ppm) and the lowest amounts in potatoes (0.01 ppm DDT) and root vegetables (carrots, beets, etc.) (0.01 ppm DDE) (Duggan et al., 1967). In garden fruits (peppers, tomatoes, etc.), a maximum value for total DDT of about 0.2 ppm has been found (Corneliussen, 1969, 1970, 1972; Duggan et al., 1966; Martin & Duggan, 1968); and in fruits, a maximum value of 0.1 ppm has been reported (Corneliussen, 1969, 1970; Duggan et al., 1967; Martin & Duggan, 1968), although up to 0.51 ppm was found by Corneliussen (1972). Small amounts of DDT have also been found in oils, grains, cereals, sugar and peanuts.

In the US, the total dietary intake decreased from 0.9 µg/kg bw DDT + DDE + TDE in 1965 to 0.4 µg/kg bw in 1970; thus the average total dietary intake for that period was 0.7 µg/kg bw (0.3 DDT, 0.2 DDE and 0.2 TDE) (Duggan & Corneliussen, 1972). Similar investigations in the UK indicate an average total DDT intake of about 0.8 µg/kg bw/day (Robinson & McGill, 1966), 0.6 µg/kg bw/day (Abbott et al., 1969) or 0.2 µg/kg bw/day (Department of Trade & Industry, 1973). In Japan, an intake of 0.5 µg/kg bw/day has been estimated (Uyeta et al., 1971).

The FAO/WHO "conditional" daily intake, which applies to DDT, DDE and TDE, singly, or in combination, is 0-0.005 mg/kg bw/day (FAO/WHO, 1970).

A threshold limit value of 1 mg/m^3 has been established in the US for an 8-hour time-weighted average occupational exposure (US Code of Federal Regulations, 1972).

2.3 Analysis

A general approach to the analysis of organochlorine pesticides has been given in the preamble (p. 16). Further analytical methods used for the detection of DDT in various media can be found in papers mentioned in the section on "Occurrence", in which actual levels are reported.

3. Biological Data Relevant to the Evaluation of Carcinogenic Risk to Man

3.1 Carcinogenicity and related studies in animals

(a) Oral administration

Mouse: In a study published as a preliminary note 18 male and 18 female (C57BL/6 x C3H/Anf)F1 mice and a similar number of (C57BL/6 x AKR)F1 mice were given single doses of 46.4 mg/kg bw p,p'-DDT by stomach tube at 7 days of age, and the same absolute amount was then given daily until the animals were 28 days of age, when they were transferred to a diet containing 140 ppm p,p'-DDT. Mice were killed at 81 weeks. In both strains, about 30% of the females died during treatment. Hepatomas were found in 11/18 male and 4/18 female (C57BL/6 x C3H/Anf)F1 mice compared with 8/79 male and 0/87 female controls, and in 7/18 male and 1/18 female (C57BL/6 x AKR)F1 mice compared with 5/90 male and 1/82 female controls. In addition, 6/18 (C57BL/6 x AKR)F1 females died with malignant lymphomas, compared to 4/82 female controls (Innes et al., 1969).

A 5-generation experiment, originally set up to investigate the effects of DDT on behaviour, was used to provide animals for a carcinogenicity study. One test and one control group of BALB/c mice were taken from each of the 5 generations and their tumour incidence studied. A total of 683 received a diet containing 3 ppm p,p'-DDT and 406 a control diet. Lung carcinomas were observed in 16.9% of the treated mice and 1.2% of the controls. (The incidence of lung adenomas is not reported, although the authors note an average incidence of 5% in their colony of mice.) The incidence of lymphomas was 4.8% in treated and 1.0% in control mice, of leukaemias 12.4% and 2.6% and of other tumours 5.8% and 1.0%, respectively (Tarján & Kemény, 1969).

A 2-generation dose-response study on the feeding of DDT to CF1 mice involving a total of 881 treated and 224 control mice has recently been reported (Tomatis et al., 1972). Dietary concentrations of 2, 10, 50 and 250 ppm technical DDT were administered for lifespan. In both the parent (P) and offspring (F1) generations there was an excess of mortality from week 60 onwards among mice receiving 250 ppm DDT. Only the incidence of liver-cell tumours was affected by exposure to DDT, and in the two sexes, it ranged as follows:

Group	male*	female*
0 ppm	25/113	4/111
2 ppm	57/124	4/105
10 ppm	52/104	11/124
50 ppm	67/127	13/104
250 ppm	82/103	69/90

(*Number of animals surviving at the time of appearance of the first tumour at any site in each group)

The excess over the controls of liver-cell tumours in mice of both sexes fed 250 ppm DDT was significant at the 1% level. The excess over the controls of liver-cell tumours in males fed 2, 10 or 50 ppm was significant at the 1% level in animals surviving more than 60 weeks. In females, all liver-cell tumours were found after 100 weeks of age, and the excess over the controls was significant at the 5% level only in the group fed 50 ppm DDT. Four liver-cell tumours, all occurring in DDT-treated mice, gave metastases. No remarkable differences were observed between P and F1 mice in this study.

These results were confirmed in a later study reporting the effect of DDT on 6 consecutive generations of CF1 mice (Turusov et al., 1973).

In a 2-generation study, a total of 515 female and 431 male BALB/c mice were administered dietary concentrations of 0, 2, 20 or 250 ppm technical DDT for lifespan. Only liver-cell tumours were found in excess, and only the 250 ppm dose level was effective. In females, the survival rates were comparable in all groups, and liver-cell tumours were found in 0/131 control mice, 0/135 mice fed 2 ppm, 1/128 mice fed 20 ppm and 71/121 mice fed 250 ppm DDT. In males, early deaths occurred in all groups as a consequence of fighting and (at the highest dosage level) because of the toxicity of DDT. In males which survived over 60 weeks of age, liver-cell tumours were found in 1/62 control mice, 3/58 receiving 2 ppm, 0/48 receiving 20 ppm and 15/31 receiving 250 ppm DDT. Liver-cell tumour distribution was unrelated to the litter of origin. No metastases were found. The tumours grew after transplantation into syngeneic animals (Terracini et al., 1973a). Confirmatory results were obtained in two subsequent generations of BALB/c mice fed DDT, although F1-F3 mice, which were exposed to DDT both in utero and after birth for lifespan developed more liver tumours than did P mice, which were exposed to DDT only after weaning (Terracini et al., 1973b).

In a multigeneration study in A strain mice, DDT in sunflower-seed oil was administered to 234 mice at doses of 10 ppm. In two control groups a total of 206 mice received either no treatment or sunflower-seed oil alone. Similar treatments were applied to the F0, F1, F2, F3, F4 and F5 generations. A further 30 mice were given doses of 0.1 ml of a 50 ppm solution which adversely affected pregnancies, thus no subsequent generations were obtained at this level. Approximately 30-50% of the animals in the treated groups died before 6 months; all animals were killed after 12 months. Only lung adenomas were found. The incidences in F0-F5 generations treated with 10 ppm DDT were as follows:-

F0, 8/42 (19%); F1, 4/26 (15%); F2, 6/25 (24%); F3, 19/41 (46%); F4, 16/37 (43%); F5, 8/63 (13%); controls (F0-F5), 15/206 (7%).

Of the 30 mice receiving 50 ppm doses, 14 died before 6 months, and 3 of these (21.5%) had lung adenomas; and of the 16 dying after this time, 8 (50%) had lung adenomas. The average number of lung nodules/mouse, about 7.2, was similar in both sexes, compared to 1.0-4.7 nodules/mouse in the 6 generations receiving 10 ppm doses and 1.0 nodule/mouse in controls (Shabad et al., 1973). (Details given in the paper are inadequate to determine the exact mode of administration of DDT in these experiments.)

Diets containing 50 or 100 ppm p,p'-DDT were administered to groups of 30-32 CF1 mice of each sex for 2 years. The control group included 47 mice of each sex. In males given 0, 50 and 100 ppm, liver tumours occurred in 13%, 37% and 53% of the animals, respectively. In females, the corresponding incidences were 17%, 50% and 76%. The ratio of liver tumours characterized by simple nodular growths of solid cords of parenchymal cells, classified as benign tumours (type a), to tumours growing with papillary or adenoid growths with cells proliferating in confluent sheets with necrosis and increased mitosis (type b) was greater than 3:1 in the treated group; no type (b) tumours occurred in controls. The incidences of other tumours were comparable in control and DDT-treated mice. Metastases were found in one treated female (Walker et al., 1973).

In a subsequent study in which 100 ppm p,p'-DDT were fed in the diet to 30 male and 30 female CF1 mice for 110 weeks, the animals were not sent for autopsy until the intra-abdominal masses reached a size which caused the animals to become anorexic or clinically affected. In this experiment, 79% of the males and 96% of the females compared with 24% and 23% in the controls developed liver tumours within 26 months. The ratio of type (a) to type (b) tumours was about 1:1 in the DDT-treated mice (Thorpe & Walker, 1973).

Rat: In two 2-year experiments started at an interval of 1 year, a total of 228 Osborne-Mendel rats received diets containing technical DDT (as a powder or as a solution in oil) at concentrations of 0 ppm (24 males and 12 females), 100 ppm (12 males), 200 ppm (24 males and 12 females), 400 ppm (24 males and 12 females), 600 ppm (24 males and 24 females) and 800 ppm (36 males and 24 females). Of the 192 rats exposed to DDT, 111 died before 18 months of treatment; only 14 rats given 800 ppm, 23 rats given 600 ppm, 14 given 400 ppm, 24 given 200 ppm, 6 given 100 ppm and 20 controls were alive at this time. Tumour incidences for each dose level are not given. Among the 81 rats surviving at least 18 months, 4 had 'low-grade' hepatic-cell carcinomas (measuring 0.5-1.2 cm) and 11 showed nodular adenomatoid hyperplasia (nodules measuring up to 0.3 cm). No liver lesions were found in control rats. Hepatic-cell tumours are reported to occur spontaneously in 1% of the rats of this colony, and nodular adenomatous hyperplasia is reported to be rare (Fitzhugh & Nelson, 1947).

DDT (the composition of which was not given) was fed to groups of 40 rats of each sex at concentrations of 0, 2.5, 12.5 and 25 ppm for 2 years. Survival rates were not affected by exposure to DDT. Only liver pathology was reported, and it was characterized by an increase of liver:body weight ratio. Tumour incidences are not reported (Treon & Cleveland, 1955).

Two experiments on Osborne-Mendel rats have been reported from the same institution, in which groups of 30 males and 30 females were exposed for at least 2 years to either 80 or 200 ppm DDT (recrystallized, purity unspecified) and compared to two control groups of 30 animals of each sex. Undifferentiated bronchogenic carcinomas were seen in 8/60 rats fed 80 ppm DDT, in 2/60 controls and in none of the animals receiving 200 ppm DDT. Two hepatomas were found in the two experiments: one occurred in a control female and the other in a female given 200 ppm DDT. Incidences of other tumours were similar in control and treated rats (Deichmann et al., 1967; Radomski et al., 1965).

A group of 15 male and 15 female Fischer rats was given doses of 10 mg/rat DDT (unspecified composition) by stomach tube, 5 times per week, starting at weaning. Treatment lasted 1 year, and survivors were observed for a further 6 months, the average survival being 14.2 months. No hepatomas were found. No data are available on the occurrence of other tumours (Weisburger & Weisburger, 1968).

(The Working Group was aware of a multigeneration study underway which will be reported shortly[1].)

Hamster: Groups of 25-30 Syrian golden hamsters of each sex were fed a diet containing either 500 or 1000 ppm p,p'-DDT in olive oil for 44 out of 48 weeks. Survivors at 50 weeks were 70/115 treated versus 59/79 control animals, and all treated animals and 62/79 controls were dead by the 90th week. Eleven treated animals developed tumours at different sites (including 1 hepatoma), as did 8 controls (Agthe et al., 1970).

Dog: A total of 22 animals approximately equally divided by sex were fed either 0 (2 dogs), 400 (2 dogs), 2000 (4 dogs) or 3200 ppm (14 dogs) DDT. Only the control dogs, the 2 dogs given 400 ppm and 2 of the dogs receiving 2000 ppm survived to the time of sacrifice (39-49 months). Liver damage but no tumours were observed (Lehman, 1952, 1965).

---

[1] IARC (1973) Annual Report 1972-1973, Lyon

Monkey: In a study, which had not been terminated at the time of reporting, dietary concentrations of either 5 or 200 ppm technical DDT were given to rhesus monkeys. Seven and a half years after the beginning of treatment 3/5 animals fed 5 ppm and 3/4 animals fed 200 ppm were alive and clinically well. In 2 additional groups of a total of 6 animals receiving 200 ppm DDT (either technical or the p,p'-isomer) 3 were alive after 3.5 years. Animals which did not survive died from intercurrent diseases (Durham et al., 1963).

Trout: A series of experiments on rainbow trout have been summarized by Halver (1967). In the first experiment a dietary concentration of 75 ppm DDT (unspecified) was fed to 30 trout for 15-20 months. Hepatomas appeared in 11 animals versus 0/400 fed the control diet. In the second experiment, dietary concentrations of either 18 or 75 ppm were given for at least 20 months. Tumour incidences were evaluated grossly through surgical inspection, and a similar excess of hepatomas was found at both dose levels. Considering both treated groups together, at 9 months after the beginning of the treatment 1/66 had a definite tumour and 4/66 had suspect lesions, versus 0/25 and 2/25 in the controls. Respective figures at later stages were: 12 months - 4 tumours and 7 suspect lesions/153 versus 1 and 6/96 in controls; 16 months - 8 tumours and 16 suspect lesions/115 versus 0 and 6/92 in controls; 20 months - 5 tumours and 15 suspect lesions/91 versus 1 and 11/71 in controls.

(b) Skin application

Mouse: A group of 14 BALB/c mice of both sexes was painted weekly with a 5% solution of DDT in kerosene for 52 weeks. A group of 16 controls received no treatment. No tumours were found (Bennison & Mostofi, 1950).

(c) Subcutaneous and/or intramuscular injection

Newborn mouse: Forty-two Swiss mice received single s.c. injections of 15,000 mg/kg bw DDT (composition unspecified) within 72 hours after birth and were killed after 6 months. Lung adenomas were not found in excess when compared with controls (Gargus et al., 1969).

3.2 Other relevant biological data[1]

(a) Metabolism and storage in animals

DDT is metabolized in a variety of mammalian species primarily by a series of alternate reductive dechlorinations and/or dehydrochlorinations (Peterson & Robison, 1964) to yield, in the first step, TDE (Klein et al., 1964) or DDE (Mattson et al., 1953; Pearce et al., 1952). As demonstrated in rats, further conversion of DDE in the liver proceeds slowly via DDMU to DDNU, while TDE is more rapidly detoxified via DDMS to DDMU to DDNU (Datta, 1970). Further metabolization of DDNU seems to occur primarily in the kidney (Datta & Nelson, 1970) to yield DDCHO via DDOH (Suggs et al., 1970) or DDA (Judah, 1949; Spicer et al., 1947). DDA is readily excreted in the urine, free or as a conjugate with cholanic acid or amino acids in the bile (Durham et al., 1963; Pinto et al., 1965).

A considerable species variation in the rates of detoxification of DDT either to TDE or DDE gives rise to variable storage levels of DDE in the adipose tissue (Durham et al., 1963; Ortega et al., 1956). A higher ratio of DDE:TDE in liver and perirenal fat after DDT administration to Swiss mice, as compared to the corresponding values in hamsters, has been reported (Gingell & Wallcave, 1974).

Conversion of DDT to TDE can also be accomplished by rat intestinal flora (Mendel & Walton, 1966).

Storage of DDT metabolites following continuous feeding

Storage levels and residues of DDT and its metabolites in CF1 and BALB/c mice given various dietary levels of technical DDT for two generations and killed 16-30 weeks after initial exposure or birth have been reported (Tomatis et al., 1971). In groups of 6-8 CF1 mice residues of

---

[1] Abbreviations used in this sub-section are as follows: DDE: 1,1-dichloro-2,2-bis(p-chlorophenyl)ethylene; TDE: 1,1-dichloro-2,2-bis(p-chlorophenyl)ethane; DDMU: 1-chloro-2,2-bis(p-chlorophenyl)ethylene; DDMS: 1-chloro-2,2-bis(p-chlorophenyl)ethane; DDNU: 2,2-bis(p-chlorophenyl)ethylene; DDOH: 2,2-bis(p-chlorophenyl)ethanol; DDCHO: 2,2-bis(p-chlorophenyl)acetaldehyde; DDA: 2,2-bis(p-chlorophenyl)acetic acid

total DDT were positively correlated with exposure levels as shown in the following table:

	Interscapular fat		Liver	
	Average (ppm)	Range	Average (ppm)	Range
controls	1.76	(1.18-2.35)	0.73	(0.18-2.09)
2 ppm	5.17	(3.05-8.15)	2.76	(0.45-15.89)
50 ppm	106.68	(53.69-220.38)	6.05	(3.41-10.52)
250 ppm	455.68	(214.83-722.19)	42.20	(19.45-86.67)

Residues of DDT in tissues of BALB/c mice given 0, 2, 20 or 250 ppm DDT were within the same range.

A comparative study with mice and hamsters has shown that following a 6-week administration of a diet containing 250 ppm p,p'-DDT, levels of total DDT in both liver and fat were 7-8 times greater in mice than in hamsters, i.e., 56-70 ppm and 8-9 ppm in mouse and hamster liver, respectively, and 2400-2500 ppm and 290-310 ppm in mouse and hamster fat, respectively; it must be taken into consideration that food consumption in mice per kg bw was 3 times greater than in hamsters. Residues present in fat as DDE represented less than 1% in both species; in the liver, DDE represented about 20% of residues in mice and 2% of residues in hamsters, the DDE:TDE ratio being about 0.5 in mice and 0.02 in hamsters (Gingell & Wallcave, 1974).

In rats, feeding of 200 ppm p,p'-DDT for 140 days led to fat concentrations of DDT in the order of 500 ppm in males and 1500 ppm in females; 10% of this was present as DDE. Concentrations in the liver of DDT and DDE were in the order of 13-25 ppm, with a DDT:DDE ratio of about 5:1 (Dale et al., 1962).

The oestrogenic effect of DDT compounds was demonstrated by Welch et al. (1969) who showed that a single dose of 50 mg/kg bw o,p'-DDT, technical DDT or p,p'-DDT produced an increase in uterine weight within 6 hours after the injection. Little or no effect was seen with o,p'-TDE, p,p'-TDE, m,p'-TDE or p,p'-DDE. After 3 daily i.p. doses of 50 mg/kg bw o,p'-TDE and m,p'-TDE, these substances were active 18 hours after the last injection. In dose-response studies, 5-10 mg/kg bw o,p'-DDT was found to be the most active. The uptake of oestradiol-17β by the rat uterus was decreased by o,p'-DDT, technical DDT or p,p'-DDT injected 2 hours before the oestradiol. DDA was also found to have oestrogenic activity in the rat (Gellert et al., 1972).

(b) Metabolism and storage in man

Ingested DDT yields, following a reductive dechlorination, TDE, which is further degraded and readily excreted in the urine as DDA (Roan et al., 1971). DDT is also slowly converted, by dehydrochlorination, into DDE (Morgan & Roan, 1971), which is retained in adipose tissue (Abbott et al., 1968; Hayes et al., 1971; Wassermann et al., 1967). No increase in the urinary excretion of DDA was noted after the oral ingestion of DDE by human volunteers, however, such an increase was observed after ingestion of TDE or DDT (Roan et al., 1971). The observations of Laws et al. (1967) of occupationally exposed people indicate that urinary levels of DDA are correlated to the levels of exposure to technical DDT and that DDT and its metabolites are stored in adipose and other tissues.

DDT is also excreted in human milk (Curley & Kimbrough, 1969; Quinby et al., 1965; Zavon et al., 1969) and transferred through the placenta (Curley et al., 1969; O'Leary et al., 1970; Zavon et al., 1969).

The ingestion of technical or p,p'-DDT during 21.5 months was studied in human volunteers. The concentration in adipose tissue after administration of technical DDT at a dose of 35 mg/man/day rose from a pre-exposure level of 4.1 ppm to 280.5 ppm after 21.5 months. After a recovery period of 37.8 months, 56.8 ppm DDT were still found to be present. The concentration of DDE amounted to 8-11% of the total DDT in adipose tissue during the dosing period; its proportional concentration relative to that of DDT increased during the recovery phase and represented 47% at the end of this period (Hayes et al., 1971). A high percentage of DDT is also stored as DDE in the general population (Durham, 1969).

Many studies on DDT and DDE storage in the adipose tissue of the general population in various countries have been reported (Abbott et al.,

1972; Curley et al., 1973; Wassermann et al., 1970, 1972a,b,c). The highest values of total DDT have been reported by Wassermann et al. (1965) in Israel (19.2 ppm, 1963-4) and the lowest in the UK (Abbott et al., 1972). In the UK the concentration of total DDT in human adipose tissue has declined from an arithmetic mean of 3.7 ppm in males and 2.7 ppm in females in 1963-64 to 2.7 ppm and 2.3 ppm, respectively, in 1969-71 (Abbott et al., 1972). A similar trend has been observed in recent years in the US (Fiserova-Bergerova et al., 1967; Morgan & Roan, 1970).

Total DDT (approximately 6-8 ppm) has been found in the adipose tissue of stillborn infants in the US (Curley et al., 1969; Fiserova-Bergerova et al., 1967; Zavon et al., 1969). Lower levels (1 ppm) have been found in stillborns in Nigeria; levels in 1-4 year olds increased to 6 ppm total DDT (Wassermann et al., 1972c).

In a population divided into three age groups, 5-25 years, 25-45 years and 45 years and above, an increase in the amount of DDT stored in body fat has been demonstrated with increase in age (Wassermann et al., 1970).

Generally, the concentration of total DDT in female human adipose tissue is lower than that in males of the general population of the same geographic area and age group (Abbott et al., 1972; Wassermann et al., 1970). For additional data on storage see table in appendix p. 224.

(c) Carcinogenicity of metabolites

TDE (DDD)

Oral administration

Mouse: In a screening study reported in a preliminary note, the carcinogenicities of o,p'-TDE and p,p'-TDE were investigated separately on groups of 18 male and 18 female (C57BL/6 x C3H/Anf)F1 and a similar number of (C57BL/6 x AKR)F1 mice. Results are not reported in detail and cannot be evaluated (Innes et al., 1969).

A group of 59 male and 59 female CF1 mice was fed a diet containing 250 ppm p,p'-TDE for lifespan, and tumour incidences were compared to those observed in a control group of 98 males and 90 females. Hepatomas were found in 52% of treated and 34% of control males and only sporadically in females. Incidences of lung tumours were 86% in males compared with 54% in controls, and 73% in females compared with 41% in controls (Tomatis et al., 1974).

Rat: A group of 10 adult male Wistar rats was fed a low-protein, low-riboflavin diet containing 600 ppm o,p'-TDE and killed at intervals from 24-469 days. Testicular damage was observed from the second month onwards. Of the 3 animals killed after 348 or more days, 1 rat had microscopical adenomatous nodules and 2 had tumours of the interstitial cells of the testes. These lesions are considered to be related to specific degenerative changes induced by o,p'-TDE on the adrenal cortex (Lacassagne & Hurst, 1965).

DDE

Oral administration

Mouse: A group of 53 male and 55 female CF1 mice was fed a diet containing 250 ppm p,p'-DDE for lifespan, and tumour incidences were compared to those observed in a control group of 98 males and 90 females. Hepatomas were found in 74% treated males and 98% treated females compared with 34% and 1% in the controls. Incidences of other tumours were not increased (Tomatis et al., 1974).

3.3 Observations in man

(a) Cross-sectional studies on workers exposed to DDT

In one study, 40 men engaged in the manufacture or formulation of DDT were medically examined. Twenty-eight of the men were under 39 years of age, 7 between 40 and 49 and 5 over 50. Twenty-four of the workers had also been exposed to other pesticides. Length of exposure at the time of the study was less than 1 year for 2 workers, 1-4 years for 21 workers and 5-8 years for 17 workers. Examination included a complete medical history, physical and neurological examinations, haemoglobin titre, white blood cell count and differential, a sulpho-bromophthalein test, plasma and erythrocyte cholinesterase determinations and measurement of urinary DDA concentration. From the latter, DDT intake was calculated for 38 workers:

it was 10-20 mg/man/day in 10 cases, around 30 mg/man/day in 15 and around 40 mg/man/day in 13. No evidence of neoplasia was found among the 40 workers at the time of investigation (Ortelee, 1958).

Another study was carried out on 35 workers with intensive occupational exposure exclusively to DDT. The group was selected from 165 persons working at the time of the study; of these only 63 had been employed for more than 5 years, and 28 of the 63 were excluded from the study for various reasons unrelated to health. Workers previously exposed to DDT but not employed at the time of the study were not included. The ages of the 35 remaining workers ranged between 30 and 63 years (mean, 43 years). The average number of years of exposure was 15 (range, 11-19). Investigations included medical histories, physical examinations, chest X-rays, blood and urine tests and measurements of fat, urine and serum concentration of DDT residues. On the basis of DDT storage and DDA excretion, the daily intake of DDT was estimated to be 3-6 mg/man in 3 workers with low exposure, 6-8 mg/man in 12 with moderate exposure and 17-18 mg/man in 20 with high exposure. No cancer was reported in any of the workers (Laws et al., 1967).

(b) Studies on volunteers

Twenty-four volunteers from a penitentiary participated in a study which started in 1956. Average age at the beginning of the study was 34 years, and exposure to DDT lasted 21.5 months. Four men were used as controls, and technical DDT was given at daily doses of 3.5 mg/man to 6 men and 35 mg/man to 6 other men. An additional group of 8 men received 35 mg/man/day p,p'-DDT. Two men in each group were kept under supervision until 4 years after the beginning of the study, and the remainder completed an additional year. No cases of tumours were recorded (Hayes et al., 1971). (This study provides no information relevant to carcinogenicity.)

(c) The concentration of DDT residues in tissues of terminal patients

Several autopsy studies have been reported attempting to correlate disease to the amounts of chlorinated hydrocarbons stored in tissues. One investigation disclosed an average concentration of total DDT and DDE in abdominal wall fat of 9.6 ± 6.5 ppm among 292 patients with cancer, compared with 9.4 ± 6.5 ppm among 396 patients with other diseases (Hoffman et al., 1967). In another study of autopsy material from 38 persons aged over 36 years, it was found that among the 19 patients with lower tissue levels of organochlorine (total DDT + dieldrin + heptachlor epoxide) 4 had malignant tumours, whereas the corresponding figure for the 19 patients with higher levels was 9 (Casarett et al., 1968). In another investigation, the average concentration of total DDT in fat tissues (unspecified) at autopsy was 21.96 ppm in 40 cases of carcinoma, 21.37 ppm in 5 cases of leukaemia, 13.66 ppm in 5 cases of Hodgkin's disease and 9.74 ppm in 42 control cases. Six patients with brain tumours had fat and brain levels of DDT residues comparable to those of the controls. In patients with non-neoplastic liver diseases, fat and liver concentrations of DDT residues were higher than in controls, although to a lesser extent than in cases of cancer with liver metastases. In all groups, high individual variations were found (Radomski et al., 1968).

(d) Case reports

Chronic liver damage (cirrhosis and chronic hepatitis) has been reported on the basis of liver biopsy in 8 workers heavily exposed to BHC, DDT or both for periods ranging from 5-13 years. Other factors such as alcoholism were reportedly excluded as the cause of the cirrhosis (Schüttmann, 1968).

4. Comments on Data Reported and Evaluation[1]

4.1 Animal data

The hepatocarcinogenicity of DDT by the oral route has been demonstrated in several strains of mice. Liver-cell tumours have been produced in both sexes, and in CF1 mice some were found to have metastasized. Increased tumour incidences have been reported in some other organs; however, this finding was not confirmed in two recent multigeneration studies using a wide range of doses.

---

[1] See also the section "Animal Data in Relation to the Evaluation of Risk to Man" in the introduction to this volume.

Oral administration studies in rats have provided no convincing evidence of carcinogenicity of DDT to this species.

In a single experiment, hamsters tolerated higher dietary intakes of DDT than did mice and rats and did not develop tumours in excess over the controls.

The negative results obtained in feeding studies with dogs and monkeys cannot be regarded as conclusive, due to limitations in group size and duration of treatment.

Liver-cell tumour induction in the trout cannot be considered as conclusive until additional studies using properly controlled diets are reported.

Skin application and subcutaneous injection studies in mice were too limited in duration and/or group size to allow any conclusions to be made.

Two dose-response studies on liver-cell tumour response to DDT following oral administration in two strains of mice are available. In both CF1 and BALB/c mice, dietary intakes of 250 ppm (corresponding to about 37.5 mg/kg bw/day) were highly effective in both sexes. The lowest dose used, 2 ppm in the diet (corresponding to an intake of about 0.3 mg/kg bw/day), induced a significant increase in the incidence of hepatomas only in male CF1 mice.

The two DDT metabolites, p,p'-DDE and TDE (DDD), were tested by oral administration to mice. The latter produced a significant increase in lung tumours, while DDE was found to produce a high incidence of liver-cell tumours.

4.2 Human data

The cross-sectional epidemiological studies on workers exposed to DDT and the observational studies on volunteers were too limited and/or too short to allow any conclusions to be made regarding carcinogenesis.

Although fat concentrations of DDT residues were higher in terminal cancer patients than in control patients, this finding is inconclusive as to a causal relationship. A similar study with a different design did not show such a result.

5. References

Abbott, D.C., Harrison, R.B., Tatton, J.O'G. & Thomson, J. (1966) Organochlorine pesticides in the atmosphere. Nature (Lond.), 211, 259

Abbott, D.C., Goulding, R. & Tatton, J.O'G. (1968) Organochlorine pesticide residues in human fat in Great Britain. Brit. med. J., iii, 146

Abbott, D.C., Holmes, D.C. & Tatton, J.O'G. (1969) Pesticide residues in the total diet in England and Wales, 1966-1967. II. Organochlorine pesticide residues in the total diet. J. Sci. Fd Agric., 20, 245

Abbott, D.C., Collins, G.B. & Goulding, R. (1972) Organochlorine pesticide residues in human fat in the United Kingdom, 1969-71. Brit. med. J., ii, 553

Adamczyk, E. (1971) DDT tolerance in some food products of animal origin. Med. Wet., 27, 690

Agthe, C., Garcia, H., Shubik, P., Tomatis, L. & Wenyon, E. (1970) Study of the potential carcinogenicity of DDT in Syrian golden hamsters. Proc. Soc. exp. Med. (N.Y.), 134, 113

Anas, R.E. & Wilson, A.J., Jr (1970) Organochlorine pesticides in fur seals. Pest. Monit. J., 3, 198

Anon. (1972a) Chemische Industrie International, 1, pp. 1-4

Anon. (1972b) Chemical Marketing Reporter, November 27, p. 5

Anon. (1972c) Chemical Industry News - India, April, p. 620

Anon. (1972d) Still hope for DDT?, Chemical Week, June 21, p. 23

Anon. (1972e) DDT's Current Uses Get General Backing of Hearing Examiner, The Wall Street Journal, April 26

Anon. (1972f) Tolerances for residues and directions for safe use of agricultural chemicals in Japan. IV. Jap. Pest. Inform., 13, 19

Anon. (1972g) Le DDT interdit en Suisse depuis le 1er avril 1972. Phytoma, 239, 37 (An English abstract is given in Health Aspects of Pesticides Abstract Bulletin, No. 72-2520)

Antommaria, P., Corn, M. & DeMaio, L. (1965) Airborne particulates in Pittsburgh: association with p,p'-DDT. Science, 150, 1476

BBLF (Biologische Bundesanstalt für Land- und Forstwirtschaft) (1972) Pflanzenschutzmittel-Verzeichnis, Merkblatt Nr. 1, 23. Auflage, April, Braunschweig, Federal Republic of Germany

Baetcke, K.P., Cain, J.D. & Poe, W.E. (1972) Mirex and DDT residues in wildlife and miscellaneous samples in Mississippi - 1970. Pest. Monit. J., 6, 14

Bennison, B.E. & Mostofi, F.K. (1950) Observations on inbred mice exposed to DDT. J. nat. Cancer Inst., 10, 989

Bergenstal, D.M., Hertz, R., Lipsett, M.B. & Moy, R.H. (1960) Chemotherapy of adrenocortical cancer with o,p'-DDD. Ann. intern. Med., 53, 672

Bevenue, A., Hylin, J.W., Kawano, Y. & Kelley, T.W. (1972) Organochlorine pesticide residues in water, sediment, algae and fish, Hawaii, 1970-71. Pest. Monit. J., 6, 56

Bledsoe, T., Roland, D.P., Hey, R.L. & Liddle, G.W. (1964) An effect of o,p'-DDD on the extra-adrenal metabolism of cortisol in man. J. clin. Endocrinol. Metabol., 24, 1303

Bjerk, J.E. & Sakshaug, J. (1969) Residues of organochlorine insecticides in samples of Norwegian butter, 1968. Nord. vet. Med., 21, 635

Bradshaw, J.S., Loveridge, E.L., Rippee, K.P., Peterson, J.L., White, D.A., Barton, J.R. & Fuhriman, D.K. (1972) Seasonal variations in residues of chlorinated hydrocarbon pesticides in the water of the Utah Lake drainage system - 1970 and 1971. Pest. Monit. J., 6, 166

Bro-Rasmussen, F., Dalgaard-Middelsen, Sv., Jakobsen, Th., Koch, Sv.O., Rodin, F., Uhl, E. & Voldum-Clausen, K. (1968) Examinations of Danish milk and butter for contaminating organochlorine insecticides. Res. Rev., 23, 55

Brown, E. & Nishioka, Y.A. (1967) Pesticides in selected western streams - a contribution to the national program. Pest. Monit. J., 1, ii, 38

Burnett, R. (1971) DDT residues: distribution of concentrations in Emerita analoga (Stimpson) along coastal California. Science, 174, 606

Casarett, L.J., Fryer, G.C., Yauger, W.L., Jr & Klemmer, H. (1968) Organochlorine pesticide residues in human tissue - Hawaii. Arch. environm. Hlth, 17, 306

Chaby Nunes, J. & Oliveira Nobre, C. (1972) Lista dos productos fitofarmacêuticos com venda autorizada, Lisbon, Secretaria de Estado da Agricultura, p. 7

Chemical Information Services Ltd. (1973) Directory of West European Chemical Producers, Oceanside, NY

Chisholm, D. & MacPhee, A.W. (1972) Persistence and effects of some pesticides in soil. J. econ. Entomol., 65, 1010

Cohen, J.M. & Pinkerton, C. (1966) Widespread translocation of pesticides by air transport and rainout. *Organic Pesticides in the Environment, Adv. Chem. Ser.*, *60*, 163

Corneliussen, P.E. (1969) Pesticide residues in total diet samples (IV). *Pest. Monit. J.*, *2*, 140

Corneliussen, P.E. (1970) Pesticide residues in total diet samples (V). *Pest. Monit. J.*, *4*, 89

Corneliussen, P.E. (1972) Pesticide residues in total diet samples (VI). *Pest. Monit. J.*, *5*, 313

Cory, L., Fjeld, P. & Serat, W. (1970) Distribution patterns of DDT residues in the Sierra Nevada Mountains. *Pest. Monit. J.*, *3*, 204

Culley, D.D. & Applegate, H.G. (1967) Insecticide concentrations in wildlife at Presidio, Texas. *Pest. Monit. J.*, *1*, ii, 21

Cummings, J.G. (1966) Pesticides in the total diet. *Res. Rev.*, *16*, 30

Cummings, J.G., Zee, K.T., Turner, V., Quinn, F. & Cook, R.E. (1966) Residues in eggs from low feeding of five chlorinated hydrocarbon insecticides in hens. *J. Ass. off. analyt. Chem.*, *49*, 354

Curley, A. & Kimbrough, R.D. (1969) Chlorinated hydrocarbon insecticides in plasma and milk of pregnant and lactating women. *Arch. environm. Hlth*, *18*, 156

Curley, A., Copeland, M.F. & Kimbrough, R.D. (1969) Chlorinated hydrocarbon insecticides in organs of stillborn and blood of newborn babies. *Arch. environm. Hlth*, *19*, 628

Curley, A., Burse, V.W., Jennings, R.W., Villanueva, E.C., Tomatis, L. & Akazaki, K. (1973) Chlorinated hydrocarbon pesticides and related compounds in adipose tissue from people of Japan. *Nature (Lond.)*, *242*, 338

Dale, W.E., Gaines, T.B. & Hayes, W.J., Jr (1962) Storage and excretion of DDT in starved rats. *Toxicol. appl. Pharmacol.*, *4*, 89

Datta, P.R. (1970) In vivo detoxication of p,p'-DDT via p,p'-DDE to p,p'-DDA in rats. In: Deichmann, W.B., Radomski, J.L. & Penalver, R.A., eds., *Pesticides Symposia. Collection of papers presented at the 6th Inter-American Conference on Toxicology and Occupational Medicine, Miami, Florida, 1968*, Miami, Florida, Halos, p. 41

Datta, P.R. & Nelson, M.J. (1970) p,p'-DDT detoxication by isolated perfused rat liver and kidney. In: Deichmann, W.B., Radomski, J.L. & Penalver, R.A., eds., *Pesticides Symposia. Collection of papers presented at the 6th Inter-American Conference on Toxicology and Occupational Medicine, Miami, Florida, 1968*, Miami, Florida, Halos, p. 47

Deichmann, W.B., Keplinger, M., Sala, F. & Glass, E. (1967) Synergism among oral carcinogens. IV. Simultaneous feeding of four tumorigens to rats. Toxicol. appl. Pharmacol., 11, 88

Department of Trade & Industry (1973) Report of the Government Chemist, 1972, London, HMSO (in press)

Deubert, K.H. & Zuckerman, B.M. (1969) Distribution of dieldrin and DDT in cranberry bog soil. Pest. Monit. J., 2, 172

Duggan, R.E. (1967) Chlorinated pesticide residues in fluid milk and other dairy products in the United States. Pest. Monit. J., 1, iii, 2

Duggan, R.E. & Corneliussen, P.E. (1972) Dietary intake of pesticide chemicals in the United States (III), June 1968-April 1970. Pest. Monit. J., 5, 331

Duggan, R.E. & Lipscomb, G.Q. (1969) Dietary intake of pesticide chemicals in the United States (II), June 1966-April 1968. Pest. Monit. J., 2, 153

Duggan, R.E. & Weatherwax, J.R. (1967) Dietary intake of pesticide chemicals. Science, 157, 1006

Duggan, R.E., Barry, H.C. & Johnson, L.Y. (1966) Pesticide residues in total diet samples. Science, 151, 101

Duggan, R.E., Barry, H.C. & Johnson, L.Y. (1967) Pesticide residues in total diet samples (II). Pest. Monit. J., 1, ii, 2

Duggan, R.E., Lipscomb, G.Q., Cox, E.L., Heatwole, R.E. & Kling, R.C. (1971) Pesticide residue levels in foods in the United States from July 1, 1963 to June 30, 1969. Pest. Monit. J., 5, 73

Durham, W.F. (1969) Body burden of pesticides in man. Ann. N.Y. Acad. Sci., 160, 183

Durham, W.F., Ortega, P. & Hayes, W.J., Jr (1963) The effect of various dietary levels of DDT on liver function, cell morphology and DDT storage in the rhesus monkey. Arch. int. Pharmacodyn., 141, 111

Durham, W.F., Armstrong, J.F. & Quinby, G.E. (1965) DDA excretion levels. Studies in persons with different degrees of exposure to DDT. Arch. environm. Hlth, 11, 76

EFOWG; EFLP; SFRA (Eidg. Forschungsanstalt für Obst-, Wein- und Gartenbau, Wädenswil; Eidg. Forschungsanstalt für landwirtschaftlichen Pflanzenbau, Zurich-Reckenholz; Station fédérale de recherches agronomiques, Lausanne) (1972) Pflanzenschutzmittel-Verzeichnis, Bern, Eidg. Drucksachen- und Materialzentrale

Earnest, R.D. & Benville, P.E., Jr (1971) Correlation of DDT and lipid levels for certain San Francisco Bay fish. Pest. Monit. J., 5, 235

Economic Documentation Office (1973) Entoma Europe, 1973-75, Hilversum, The Netherlands

Edmundson, W.F., Davies, J.E., Nachman, G.A. & Roeth, R.L. (1969) p,p'-DDT and p,p'-DDE in blood samples of occupationally exposed workers. Publ. Hlth Rep. (Wash.), 84, 53

Edwards, C.A. (1966) Insecticide residues in soils. Res. Rev., 13, 83

Egan, H., Goulding, R., Roburn, J. & Tatton, J.O'G. (1965) Organochlorine pesticide residues in human fat and human milk. Brit. med. J., iii, 66

Egan, H., Holmes, D.C., Roburn, J. & Tatton, J.O'G. (1966) Pesticide residues in foodstuffs in Great Britain. II. Persistent organochlorine pesticide residues in selected foods. J. Sci. Fd Agric., 17, 563

Engst, R. & Knoll, R. (1971) DDT- und DDE-Rückstände in Humanmilch. Ernährungsforsch., 16, 569

FAO (1972) FAO Production Yearbook - 1971, 25, Rome, p. 499

FAO/WHO (1967) Evaluation of some pesticide residues in food. FAO/PL: CP/15; WHO/Food Add./67.32

FAO/WHO (1968) 1967 Evaluations of some pesticide residues in food. FAO/PL:1967/M/11/1; WHO/Food Add./68.30, p. 9

FAO/WHO (1969) 1968 Evaluations of some pesticide residues in food. FAO/PL/1968/M/9/1; WHO/Food Add./69.35

FAO/WHO (1970) 1969 Evaluations of some pesticide residues in food. FAO/PL/1969/M/17/11; WHO/Food Add./70.38, p. 63

FAO/WHO (1973) Pesticide residues in food. Report of the 1972 Joint FAO/WHO Meeting. Wld Hlth Org. techn. Rep. Ser., No. 525, pp. 30, 31

Faust, S.D., ed. (1972) Fate of Organic Pesticides in the Aquatic Environment. A symposium sponsored by the Division of Pesticide Chemistry at the 161st meeting of the American Chemical Society, Los Angeles, 1971, Adv. Chem. Series 111, Washington DC, American Chemical Society

Finkelstein, H. (1969) Preliminary air pollution survey of pesticides, a literature review. Raleigh, NC, US Department of Health Education and Welfare, National Air Pollution Control Administration

Fiserova-Bergerova, V., Radomski, J.L., Davies, J.E. & Davis, J.H. (1967) Levels of chlorinated hydrocarbon pesticides in human tissues. Industr. Med. Surg., 36, 65

Fitzhugh, O.G. & Nelson, A.A. (1947) The chronic oral toxicity of DDT (2,2-bis(p-chlorophenyl)-1,1,1-trichloroethane). J. Pharmacol. exp. Ther., 89, 18

Frank, R., Braun, H.E. & McWade, J.W. (1970) Chlorinated hydrocarbon residues in the milk supply of Ontario, Canada. Pest. Monit. J., 4, 31

Gallagher, T.F., Fukushima, D.K. & Hellmann, L. (1962) The effect of ortho, para DDD on steroid borne metabolites in adrenocortical carcinoma. Metabol. clin. Exp., 11, 1155

Gargus, J.L., Paynter, O.E. & Reese, W.H., Jr (1969) Utilization of newborn mice in the bioassay of chemical carcinogens. Toxicol. appl. Pharmacol., 15, 552

Gellert, R.J., Heinrichs, W.L. & Swerdloff, R.S. (1972) DDT homologues: estrogen-like effects on the vagina, uterus and pituitary of the rat. Endocrinol., 91, 1095

Gingell, R. & Wallcave, L. (1974) Comparative studies of the acute toxicity and tissue distribution of DDT in mice and hamsters. Toxicol. appl. Pharmacol. (in press)

Hagyard, S.B., Brown, W.H., Stull, J.W., Whiting, F.M. & Kemberling, S.R. (1973) DDT and DDE content of human milk in Arizona. Bull. environm. contam. Toxicol., 9, 169

Halver, J.E. (1967) Crystalline aflatoxin and other vectors for trout hepatoma. In: Halver, J.E. & Mitchell, I.A., eds., Trout Hepatoma Research Conference Papers. Bureau of Sport Fisheries and Wild Life Research Rep. No. 70, Washington DC, Department of the Interior, p. 78

Hayashi, M. (1971) Residues of agricultural drugs and health of children. Shohni Hoken Kenkyu (Children Hlth Study), 30, 1

Hayes, W.J., Jr (1959) Pharmacology and toxicology of DDT. In: Müller, P., ed., DDT: The insecticide dichlorodiphenyltrichloroethane and its significance, 2, Basel, Birkhäuser Verlag, p. 2

Hayes, W.J. Jr, Durham, W.F. & Cueto, C., Jr (1956) The effect of known repeated oral doses of chlorophenothane (DDT) in man. J. amer. med. Ass., 162, 890

Hayes, W.J. Jr, Dale, W.E. & Pirkle, C.I. (1971) Evidence of safety of long-term, high, oral doses of DDT for man. Arch. environm. Hlth, 22, 119

Henderson, C., Inglis, A. & Johnson, W.L. (1971) Organochlorine insecticide residues in fish - fall 1969, national pesticide monitoring program. Pest. Monit. J., 5, 1

Herzel, F. (1972) Organochlorine insecticides in surface waters in Germany - 1970 and 1971. Pest. Monit. J., 6, 179

Heyndrickx, A. & Maes, R. (1969) The excretion of chlorinated hydrocarbon insecticides in human mother milk. J. Pharm. belg., 24, 459

Hoffman, W.S., Adler, H., Fishbein, W.I. & Bauer, F.C. (1967) Relation of pesticide concentrations in fat to pathological changes in tissues. Arch. environm. Hlth, 15, 758

Innes, J.R.M., Ulland, B.M., Valerio, M.G., Petrucelli, L., Fishbein, L., Hart, E.R., Pallotta, A.J., Bates, R.R., Falk, H.L., Gart, J.J., Klein, M., Mitchell, I. & Peters, J. (1969) Bioassay of pesticides and industrial chemicals for tumorigenicity in mice. A preliminary note. J. nat. Cancer Inst., 42, 1101

Johnson, D.W. & Lew, S. (1970) Chlorinated hydrocarbon pesticides in representative fishes of Southern Arizona. Pest. Monit. J., 4, 57

Johnson, L.G. & Morris, R.L. (1971) Chlorinated hydrocarbon pesticides in Iowa rivers. Pest. Monit. J., 4, 216

Judah, J.D. (1949) Studies on the metabolism and mode of action of DDT. Brit. J. Pharmacol., 4, 120

Klein, A.K., Laug, E.P., Datta, P.R., Watts, J.O. & Chen, J.T. (1964) Metabolites: reductive dechlorination of DDT to DDD and isomeric transformation of o,p'-DDT to p,p'-DDT in vivo. J. Ass. off. analyt. Chem., 47, 1129

Kroger, M. (1972) Insecticide residues in human milk. J. Pediat., 80, 401

Lacassagne, A. & Hurst, L. (1965) Les tumeurs expérimentales de la glande interstitielle du rat à propos d'une manifestation oncogénique de l'o,p'-dichlorodiphényldichloroéthane sur le testicule. Bull. Cancer, 52, 89

Laug, E.P., Kunze, F.M. & Prickett, C.S. (1951) Occurrence of DDT in human fat and milk. Arch. industr. Hyg., 3, 245

Läuger, von P., Martin, H. & Müller, P. (1944) Über Konstitution und toxische Wirkung von natürlichen und neuen synthetischen insektentötenden Stoffen. Helv. chim. Acta, 27, 892

Lawless, E.W., Rumker, R. & Ferguson, T.L. (1972) *The Pollution Potential in Pesticide Manufacturing, Pesticide Study Series-5*, Technical Studies Report TS-00-72-04, Environmental Protection Agency, Washington DC, US Government Printing Office

Laws, E.R., Jr, Curley, A. & Biros, F.J. (1967) Men with intensive occupational exposure to DDT. A clinical and chemical study. *Arch. environm. Hlth*, 15, 766

Le Boeuf, B.J. & Bonnell, M.L. (1971) DDT in California sea lions. *Nature (Lond.)*, 234, 108

Lehman, A.J. (1952) Chemicals in foods - a report to the association of food and drug officials on current developments. II. Pesticides. III. Subacute and chronic toxicity. *Quarterly Bull. Ass. F. & D. Officials of US*, 16, 47

Lehman, A.J., ed. (1965) *DDT (a mixture of 1,1,1-trichloro-2,2-bis(p-chlorophenyl)ethane and 1,1,1-trichloro-2-(o-chlorophenyl)-2-(p-chlorophenyl)ethane)*. In: *Summaries of pesticide toxicity*, Food & Drug Administration, US Department of Health, Education & Welfare, Washington DC, US Government Printing Office, p. 17

Lichtenberg, J.L., Eichelberger, J.W., Dressman, R.C. & Longbottom, J.E. (1970) Pesticides in surface waters of the United States - a 5-year summary, 1964-68. *Pest. Monit. J.*, 4, 71

Manigold, D.B. & Schulze, J.A. (1969) Pesticides in selected western streams - a progress report. *Pest. Monit. J.*, 3, 124

Martin, H., ed. (1971) *Pesticide Manual. Basic Information on the Chemicals used as Active Components of Pesticides*, 2nd ed., Ombersley, British Crop Protection Council, p. 428

Martin, R.J. & Duggan, R.E. (1968) Pesticide residues in total diet samples (III). *Pest. Monit. J.*, 1, iv, 11

Mattson, A.M., Spillane, J.T., Baker, C. & Pearce, G.W. (1953) Determination of DDT and related substances in human fat. *Analyt. Chem.*, 25, 1065

McCaskill, W.R., Phillips, B.H., Jr & Thomas, C.A. (1970) Residues of chlorinated hydrocarbons in soybean seed and surface soils from selected counties of South Carolina. *Pest. Monit. J.*, 4, 42

McGill, A.E. & Robinson, J. (1968) Organochlorine insecticide residues in complete prepared meals: a 12-month survey in SE England. *Fd Cosmet. Toxicol.*, 6, 45

Melnikov, N.N. & Schevchenko, M.G. (1971) Hygienic normalization of pesticide residues and their tolerance levels in foodstuffs in the USSR. *Res. Rev.*, 35, 1

Mendel, J.L. & Walton, M.S. (1966) Conversion of p,p'-DDT to p,p'-DDD by intestinal flora of the rat. Science, 151, 1527

Metcalf, R.L. (1966) Insecticides. In: Kirk, R.E. & Othmer, D.F., eds, Encyclopedia of Chemical Technology, 2nd ed., New York, John Wiley & Sons, Vol. 11, p. 677

Morgan, D.P. & Roan, C.C. (1970) Chlorinated hydrocarbon pesticide residues in human tissues. Arch. environm. Hlth, 20, 452

Morgan, D.P. & Roan, C.C. (1971) Absorption, storage and metabolic conversion of ingested DDT and DDT metabolites in man. Arch. environm. Hlth, 22, 301

O'Leary, J.A., Davies, J.E., Edmundson, W.F. & Reich, G.A. (1970) Transplacental passage of pesticides. Am. J. Obstet. Gynecol., 107, 65

Ortega, P., Hayes, W.J., Jr, Durham, W.F. & Mattson, A. (1956) DDT in the diet of the rat. Its effect on DDT storage, liver function and cell morphology. Publ. Hlth Monogr. No. 43, Washington DC, US Government Printing Office, p. 1

Ortelee, M.F. (1958) Study of men with prolonged intensive occupational exposure to DDT. Arch. industr. Hlth, 18, 433

Pearce, G.W., Mattson, A.M. & Hayes, W.J., Jr (1952) Examination of human fat for the presence of DDT. Science, 116, 254

Peterle, T.J. (1969) DDT in antarctic snow. Nature (Lond.), 224, 620

Peterson, J.E. & Robison, W.H. (1964) Metabolic products of p,p'-DDT in the rat. Toxicol. appl. Pharmacol., 6, 321

Pinto, J.D., Camien, M.N. & Dunn, M.S. (1965) Metabolic fate of p,p'-DDT (1,1,1-trichloro-2,2-bis(p-chlorophenyl)ethane) in rats. J. biol. Chem., 240, 2148

Prospero, J.M. & Seba, D.B. (1972) Some additional measurements of pesticides in the lower atmosphere of the northern equatorial Atlantic Ocean. Atmosph. Environm., 6, 363

Quinby, G.E., Armstrong, J.F. & Durham, W.F. (1965) DDT in human milk. Nature (Lond.), 207, 726

Radomski, J.L., Deichmann, W.B., MacDonald, W.E. & Glass, E.M. (1965) Synergism among oral carcinogens. I. Results of simultaneous feeding of four tumorigens to rats. Toxicol. appl. Pharmacol., 7, 652

Radomski, J.L., Deichmann, W.B. & Clizer, E.E. (1968) Pesticide concentrations in the liver, brain and adipose tissue of terminal hospital patients. Fd Cosmet. Toxicol., 6, 209

Ragno, M., ed. (1972) *Repertorio Chimico Italiano, Industriale e Commerciale,* Milano, Asiminum

Reinert, R.E. (1970) Pesticide concentrations in Great Lakes fish. *Pest. Monit. J.*, 3, 233

Risebrough, R.W., Huggett, R.J., Griffin, J.J. & Goldberg, E.D. (1968) Pesticides: transatlantic movements in the northeast trades. *Science,* 159, 1233

Roan, C.C., Morgan, D.P. & Paschal, E. (1971) Urinary excretion of DDA following ingestion of DDT and DDT metabolites in man. *Arch. environm. Hlth,* 22, 309

Robinson, J. & McGill, A.E.J. (1966) Organochlorine insecticide residues in complete prepared meals in Great Britain during 1965. *Nature (Lond.),* 212, 1037

Saha, J.G. (1969) Significance of organochlorine insecticide residues in fresh plants as possible contaminants of milk and beef products. *Res. Rev.*, 26, 89

Saha, J.G. & Sumner, A.K. (1971) Organochlorine insecticide residues in soil from vegetable farms in Saskatchewan. *Pest. Monit. J.*, 5, 28

Sand, P.F., Wiersma, G.B. & Landry, J.L. (1972) Pesticide residues in sweet potatoes and soil - 1969. *Pest. Monit. J.*, 5, 342

Schorr, B. (1972) Agency is likely to ban most uses of DDT in US today; foreign lands may follow. *The Wall Street Journal,* June 14, p. 30

Schüttmann, U. (1968) Chronische Lebererkrankungen nach beruflicher Einwirkung von Dichlordiphenyltrichloräthan (DDT) und Hexachlorcyclohexan (HCH). *Int. Arch. Gewerbepath. Gewerbehyg.*, 24, 193

Seal, W.L., Dawsey, L.H. & Cavin, G.E. (1967) Monitoring for chlorinated hydrocarbon pesticides in soil and root crops in the eastern states in 1965. *Pest. Monit. J.*, 1, iii, 22

Seba, D.B. & Prospero, J.M. (1971) Pesticides in the lower atmosphere of the northern equatorial Atlantic ocean. *Atmosph. Environm.*, 5, 1043

Shabad, L.M., Kolesnichenko, T.S. & Nikonova, T.V. (1973) Transplacental and combined long-term effect of DDT in five generations of A-strain mice. *Int. J. Cancer,* 11, 688

Southern, A.L., Tochimoto, S., Isurugi, K., Gorcher, G.G., Krikun, E. & Stypulkowski, W. (1966a) The effect of 2,2-bis-(2-chlorophenyl-5-chlorophenyl)-1,1-dichloro-ethane (o,p'-DDD) on the metabolism of infused cortisol-7-H. *Steroids,* 7, 11

Southern, A.L., Tochimoto, S., Strom, L., Ratuschni, A., Rass, H. & Gorcher, G. (1966b) Remission in Cushing's syndrome with o,p'-DDD. J. clin. Endocrinol. Metabol., 26, 268

Spicer, S.S., Sweeney, T.R., Oettingen, W.F., Lillie, R.D. & Neal, P.A. (1947) Toxicological observations on goats fed larger doses of DDT. Vet. Rec., 42, 289

Stanley, C.R., Barney, J.E., II, Helton, M.R. & Yobs, A.R. (1971) Measurement of atmospheric levels of pesticides. Environm. Sci. Technol., 5, 430

Stenersen, J. (1972) Pesticides for plant protection in Norway: legislation, use and residues. Res. Rev., 42, 91

Stenersen, J. & Friestad, H.O. (1969) Residues of DDT and DDE in soil from Norwegian fruit orchards. Acta agric. scand., 19, 240

Suggs, J.E., Hawk, R.E., Curley, A., Boozer, E.L. & McKinney, J.D. (1970) DDT metabolism: oxidation of the metabolite 2,2-bis(p-chlorophenyl) ethanol by alcohol dehydrogenase. Science, 168, 582

Tabor, E.C. (1965) Pesticides in urban atmospheres. J. air Pollut. Control Ass., 15, 415

Tabor, E.C. (1966) Contamination of urban air through the use of insecticides. Trans. N.Y. Acad. Sci., 28, 569.

Tarján, R. & Kemény, T. (1969) Multigeneration studies on DDT in mice. Fd Cosmet. Toxicol., 7, 215

Terracini, B., Testa, M.C., Cabral, J.R. & Day, N. (1973a) The effects of long-term feeding of DDT to BALB/c mice. Int. J. Cancer, 11, 747

Terracini, B., Cabral, R.J. & Testa, M.C. (1973b) A multigeneration study on the effects of continuous administration of DDT to BALB/c mice. In: Deichmann, W.B., ed., Proceedings of the 8th Inter-American Conference on Toxicology: Pesticides and the environment, a continuing controversy. Miami, Florida, 1973, New York, London, Intercontinental Medical Book Corp., p. 77

Thorpe, E. & Walker, A.I.T. (1973) The toxicology of dieldrin (HEOD). II. Comparative long-term oral toxicity studies in mice with dieldrin, DDT, phenobarbitone, β-BHC and γ-BHC. Fd Cosmet. Toxicol., 11, 433

Tolle, A., Heeschen, W. & Bluethgen, A. (1972) Chlorierte Insektizide, Fasziolizide und Antibiotika in der Milch. Ber. Landwirt., 50, 720

Tomatis, L., Turusov, V., Terracini, B., Day, N., Barthel, W.F., Charles, R.T., Collins, G.B. & Boiocchi, M. (1971) Storage levels of DDT metabolites in mouse tissues following long-term exposure to technical DDT. Tumori, 57, 377

Tomatis, L., Turusov, V., Day, N. & Charles, R.T. (1972) The effect of long-term exposure to DDT on CF-1 mice. Int. J. Cancer, 10, 489

Tomatis, L., Turusov, V., Charles, R.T. & Boiocchi, M. (1974) The effect of long-term exposure to 1,1-dichloro-2,2-bis(p-chlorophenyl)ethylene (p,p'-DDE), to 1,1-dichloro-2,2-bis(p-chlorophenyl)ethane (p,p'-DDD) and to the two chemicals combined, on CF-1 mice. J. nat. Cancer Inst., 52 (in press)

Trautmann, W.L., Chesters, G. & Pionke, H.B. (1968) Organochlorine insecticide composition of randomly selected soils from nine states - 1967. Pest. Monit. J., 2, 93

Treon, J.F. & Cleveland, F.P. (1955) Toxicity of certain chlorinated hydrocarbon insecticides for laboratory animals with special reference to aldrin and dieldrin. J. agric. Fd Chem., 3, 402

Turusov, V.S., Day, N.E., Tomatis, L., Gati, E. & Charles, R.T. (1973) Tumors in CF-1 mice exposed for six consecutive generations to DDT. J. nat. Cancer Inst., 51, 983

Uhnak, J. (1971) DDT and other chlorinated insecticides in milk. Vyziva Zdravie, 16, 21

UK Ministry of Agriculture, Fisheries & Food (1973) List of approved products and their uses for farmers and growers, London, pp. 82-84

US Bureau of the Census (1973) US Exports, FT 410, December 1972, Washington DC, US Government Printing Office

US Code of Federal Regulations (1972) Washington DC, US Government Printing Office, 29 CFR 1910.93, p. 46

US Department of Commerce (1970) Chemicals, June, p. 19

US Department of Commerce (1972) Chemicals, December 1971/March 1972, Washington DC, US Government Printing Office, p. 31

US Department of Health, Education & Welfare (1969) Report of the Secretary's Commission on Pesticides and their Relationship to Environmental Health, Washington DC, US Government Printing Office

US Environmental Protection Agency (1973) Water pollution prevention and control. Proposed list of toxic pollutants, US Federal Register, 38, No. 129, Washington DC, US Government Printing Office, p. 18044

US Tariff Commission (1964) Synthetic Organic Chemicals, United States Production and Sales, 1963, TC Publication 143, Washington DC, US Government Printing Office, p. 52

US Tariff Commission (1971) Synthetic Organic Chemicals, United States Production and Sales, 1969, TC Publication 412, Washington DC, US Government Printing Office, p. 190

US Tariff Commission (1973) Imports of Benzenoid Chemicals and Products, 1972, TC Publication 601, Washington DC, US Government Printing Office, p. 94

Uyeta, M., Taue, S., Chikazawa, K. & Nishimoto, T. (1971) Pesticides translocated in food - organochlorine pesticides in the total diet. Shokuhin Eiseigaku Zasshi (J. Fd Hyg. Soc. Jap.), 12, 445

Verdon, T.A., Jr, Binton, J., Herman, R.H. & Beisel, W.R. (1962) Clinical and chemical response of functioning adrenalcortical carcinoma to ortho, para-DDD. Metab. clin. Exp., 11, 226

Walker, A.I.T., Thorpe, E. & Stevenson, D.E. (1973) The toxicology of dieldrin (HEOD). I. Long-term oral toxicity studies in mice. Fd Cosmet. Toxicol., 11, 415

Wallace, Z.E., Silverstone, J.N., Vulladolid, L.S. & Weisenfeld, S. (1961) Cushing's syndrome due to adrenocortical hyperplasia. New Engl. J. Med., 265, 1088

Ware, G.W., Estesen, B.J. & Cahill, W.P. (1968) An ecological study of DDT residues in Arizona soils and alfalfa. Pest. Monit. J., 2, 129

Wassermann, M., Iliescu, S., Mandric, G. & Horvath, P. (1960) Toxic hazards during DDT- and BHC-spraying of forests against Lymantria monacha. Arch. industr. Hlth, 21, 503

Wassermann, M., Gon, M., Wassermann, D. & Zellermayer, L. (1965) DDT and DDE in the body fat of people in Israel. Arch. environm. Hlth, 11, 375

Wassermann, M., Wassermann, D., Zellermayer, L. & Gon, M. (1967) Storage of DDT in the people of Israel. Pest. Monit. J., 2, 15

Wassermann, M., Wassermann, D. & Lazarovici, S. (1970) Present state of the storage of the organochlorine insecticides in the general population of South Africa. South Afr. Med. J., 44, 646

Wassermann, M., Nogueira, D.P., Tomatis, L., Athie, E., Wassermann, D., Djavaherian, M. & Guttel, C. (1972a) Storage of organochlorine insecticides in people of Sao Paulo, Brazil. Industr. Med., 41, 22

Wassermann, M., Rogoff, M.G., Tomatis, L., Day, N.E., Wassermann, D., Djavaherian, M. & Guttel, C. (1972b) Storage of organochlorine insecticides in the adipose tissue of people in Kenya. Ann. Soc. belge Méd. trop., 52, 509

Wassermann, M., Sofoluwe, G.O., Tomatis, L., Day, N.E., Wassermann, D. & Lazarovici, S. (1972c) Storage of organochlorine insecticides in people of Nigeria. Environm. Physiol. Biochem., 2, 59

Weisburger, J.H. & Weisburger, E.K. (1968) Food additives and chemical carcinogens: on the concept of zero tolerance. Fd Cosmet. Toxicol., 6, 235

Welch, R.M., Levin, W. & Conney, A.H. (1969) Estrogenic action of DDT and its analogs. Toxicol. appl. Pharmacol., 14, 358

Wheatley, G.A. & Hardman, J.A. (1965) Indications of the presence of organochlorine insecticides in rainwater in central England. Nature (Lond.), 207, 486

Wiemeyer, S.N., Mulhern, B.M., Ligas, F.J., Hensel, R.L., Mathisen, J.E., Robards, F.C. & Postupalsky, S. (1972) Residues of organochlorine pesticides, polychlorinated biphenyls and mercury in bald eagle eggs and changes in shell thickness - 1969 and 1970. Pest. Monit. J., 6, 50

Wiersma, G.B., Taï, H. & Sand, P.F. (1972a) Pesticide residues in soil from eight cities - 1969. Pest. Monit. J., 6, 126

Wiersma, G.B., Mitchell, W.G. & Stanford, C.L. (1972b) Pesticide residues in onions and soil - 1969. Pest. Monit. J., 5, 345

Wolfe, H.R. & Armstrong, J.F. (1971) Exposure of formulating plant workers to DDT. Arch. environm. Hlth, 23, 169

Wolfe, H.R., Walker, K.C., Elliott, J.W. & Durham, W.F. (1959) Evaluation of the health hazards involved in house-spraying with DDT. Bull. Wld Hlth Org., 20, 1

Wolfe, H.R., Durham, W.F. & Armstrong, J.F. (1967) Exposure of workers to pesticides. Arch. environm. Hlth, 14, 622

Wolman, A.A. & Wilson, A.J., Jr (1970) Occurrence of pesticides in whales. Pest. Monit. J., 4, 8

Wolter, D. (1972) DDT in Oberflächengewässern. Z. gesamte Hyg., 18, 247

Wolter, D. & Rugenstein, H. (1971) DDT in Oberflächengewässern. Z. gesamte Hyg., 17, 264

Woodwell, G.M., Craig, P.P. & Johnson, H.A. (1971) DDT in the biosphere: where does it go? Science, 174, 1101

Wright, F.C., Riner, J.C. & Younger, R.L. (1972) Residues in chickens given DDT. J. agric. Fd Chem., 20, 17

Zavon, M.R., Tye, R. & Latorre, L. (1969) Chlorinated hydrocarbon insecticide content of the neonate. <u>Ann. N.Y. Acad. Sci.</u>, <u>160</u>, 196

DIELDRIN

Dieldrin is the common name approved by the International Standards Organization (except in Canada, Denmark and USSR) for a material containing not less than 85% of 1,2,3,4,10,10-hexachloro-6,7-epoxy-1,4,4a,5,6,7,8,8a-octahydro-exo-1,4-endo-5,8-dimethanonaphthalene. In Canada, dieldrin refers to the pure compound, which is known in Great Britain as HEOD. Several reviews on this compound are available (FAO/WHO, 1967, 1968, 1969, 1970, 1971).

1. Chemical and Physical Data

1.1 Synonyms and trade names

Chem. Abstr. No.: 60-57-1

Compound 497; endo-exo isomer of 1,2,3,4,10,10-hexachloro-6,7-epoxy-1,4,4a,5,6,7,8,8a-octahydro-1,4,5,8-dimethanonaphthalene; ENT 16,225; HEOD; 1,2,3,4,10,10-hexachloro-6,7-epoxy-1,4,4a,5,6,7,8,8a-octahydro-endo-exo-1,4:5,8-dimethanonaphthalene; 1,2,3,4,10,10-hexachloro-6,7-epoxy-1,4,4a,5,6,7,8,8a-octahydro-endo-1,4-exo-5,8-dimethanonaphthalene; 1,2,3,4,10,10-hexachloro-6,7-epoxy-1,4,4a,5,6,7,8,8a-octahydro-1,4-endo-exo-5,8-dimethanonaphthalene; 1,2,3,4,10,10-hexachloro-6,7-epoxy-1,4,4a,5,6,7,8,8a-octahydro-1,4-endo,exo-5,8-dimethanonaphthalene; 1,2,3,4,10,10-hexachloro-6,7-epoxy-1,4,4a,5,6,7,8,8a-octahydro-exo-1,4-endo-5,8-dimethanonaphthalene; 1,2,3,4,10,10-hexachloro-6,7-epoxy-1,4,4a,5,6,7,8,8a-octahydro-1,4-exo-5,8-endo-dimethanonaphthalene

1.2 Chemical formula and molecular weight

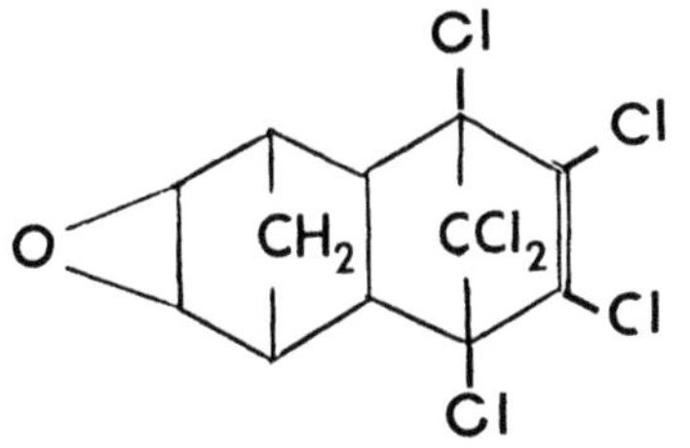

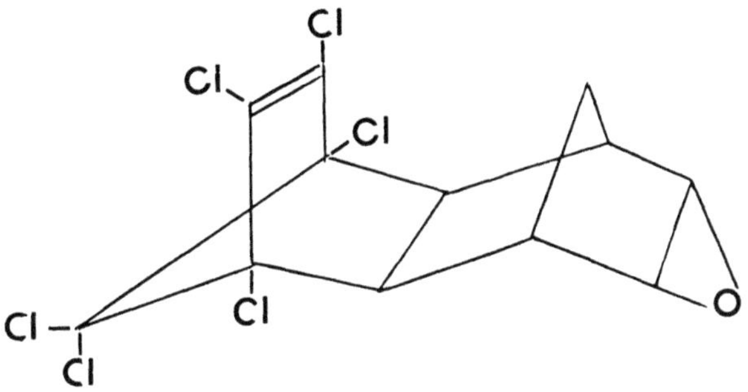

$C_{12}H_8Cl_6O$
Mol. wt: 380.9

1.3 Chemical and physical properties of the pure substance (HEOD)

(a) Description: White, odourless crystals

(b) Melting-point: 176-177°C

(c) Solubility: Practically insoluble in water (0.186 mg/l at 25-29°C); slightly soluble in petroleum oils; moderately soluble in acetone; soluble in aromatic solvents

(d) Volatility: Vapour pressure is 1.78×10^{-7} mm Hg at 20°C

(e) Chemical reactivity: Dieldrin is stable in alkalis and in acids except for strong mineral acids. Of the various compounds that can be produced by sunlight, photodieldrin is the only product of any established importance (Rosen et al., 1966; Robinson et al., 1966)

1.4 Technical products and impurities

Dieldrin is available in the United States as a technical grade product containing 100% active ingredient (equivalent to 85% of HEOD and 15% of other insecticidally-active, related compounds) with 55-56% chlorine content, less than 0.4% free acid (as HCl) and less than 0.1% water (Frear, 1972; Whetstone, 1964). It is formulated into emulsifiable concentrates, solutions, wettable powders, dusts, granules and mixtures with fertilizers.

2. Production, Use, Occurrence and Analysis

Two review articles on dieldrin have appeared (Galley, 1970; Whetstone, 1964).

2.1 Production and use[1]

Dieldrin was first synthesized in the laboratory in 1948 (Galley, 1970), and commercial production in the US was first reported in 1950 (US Tariff Commission, 1951). Dieldrin is believed to be made commercially by the epoxidation of aldrin with a peracid (e.g., peracetic or perbenzoic acid),

---

[1] Data from Chemical Information Services, Stanford Research Institute, USA

but it can also be made by the condensation of hexachlorocyclopentadiene with the epoxide of bicycloheptadiene (Galley, 1970).

Only one company in the US manufactures dieldrin, and Whetstone (1964) has estimated that this manufacturer sold 2.3-4.5 million kg of the product in 1962. Another source has estimated that less than 450 thousand kg of dieldrin were produced in 1971 (Johnson, 1972).

Imports of dieldrin through the principal US customs districts were reported to have been nearly 6 thousand kg in 1969 (US Tariff Commission, 1970) and 57 thousand kg in 1972 (US Tariff Commission, 1973).

The following European countries were reported to be producing dieldrin in 1972 or 1973 (the number of producing companies is given in parentheses): Belgium (1), France (1), Italy (2), The Netherlands (1) and the United Kingdom (1) (Chemical Information Services Ltd., 1973; Economic Documentation Office, 1973; Ragno, 1972). In 1972, Japan was reported to have had 8 suppliers of dieldrin and dieldrin formulations, some of which may also be producers of dieldrin (Chemical Daily Co., 1973), and imports into that country were reported to have been 42 thousand kg in 1970 (Hayashi, 1971).

The quantities of this material used in, or sold for agricultural uses in 1970 were reported to have been as follows (thousand kg): Colombia (27.8); El Salvador (2.6); Ghana (0.5); Israel (1.0); Italy (9.7); Madagascar (0.1); The Republic of Khmer (0.3); Sudan (4.5); and Uruguay (10.0) (FAO, 1972).

The only known use for dieldrin is as an insecticide, and one significant outlet is in the treatment of soil around structures for the control of termites, although the less expensive related pesticide, aldrin, may have dominated this market in the past. In 1972, one source estimated that 80% of the combined US production of aldrin and dieldrin was used on corn crops and about 10% for termite control (Anon., 1972a). Dieldrin is used in the US for mothproofing woollen clothes and carpets (Lipson, 1970), but the quantity consumed in this way is believed to be quite small, and such uses are now restricted to operations where there is no effluent discharge

(US Environmental Protection Agency, 1973a). It is widely used elsewhere for the same purpose, but the amounts consumed are unknown.

As of February 15, 1973 dieldrin was approved in the US for use on 46 agricultural crops (including several types of seeds) and for soil treatment around certain fruits, grains, nuts and vegetables. Tolerances for residues of dieldrin were set at 0-0.1 mg/kg on many raw agricultural products, and restrictions were placed on the use of treated seeds. Dieldrin was also approved for use as an insecticide on sheep, in barns (excluding dairy barns and poultry houses), in open-range poultry houses and for control of imported fire ants and red harvest ants (US Environmental Protection Agency, 1973b). The approved uses for dieldrin have been reviewed by the controlling US government agencies several times in the last few years because of its persistence in the environment, and recently the manufacturer voluntarily withdrew dieldrin from a number of the approved uses, e.g., imported fire ant control (US Environmental Protection Agency, 1973a). The latest of these governmental reviews was still in progress in October 1973.

Dieldrin usage in California, a major agricultural state, was reported to have been nearly 32 thousand kg in 1971 (California Department of Agriculture, 1972), and nearly 37 thousand kg in 1972 (34% of this was for control of insects in structures, 14% was used on grapes and 13% was used on pears) (California Department of Agriculture, 1973).

On July 3, 1973 the US Environmental Protection Agency proposed a list of toxic pollutants, which includes dieldrin (US Environmental Protection Agency, 1973c). If this list is adopted, effluent standards restricting or prohibiting discharges of dieldrin into streams may come into effect.

An indication of the possible uses of dieldrin can be derived from the FAO/WHO recommended residue limits for dieldrin on the following food products: asparagus, broccoli, Brussels sprouts, cabbages, cauliflowers, cucumbers, aubergines, horseradishes, onions, parsnips, peppers, pimentoes, radishes, radish tops, fruit (citrus and other), rice, potatoes, carrots, lettuces, milk and milk products, raw cereals and eggs (FAO/WHO, 1973).

The use of dieldrin has been banned in Japan (Ogata, 1972) and Switzerland (Anon., 1972b), and its sale is permitted neither in the Federal Republic of Germany nor in Italy.

2.2 Occurrence

(a) Occupational exposure

The intake by occupationally exposed workers has been estimated to range from 0.72-1.10 mg/man/day (Hayes & Curley, 1968), compared to 0.025 mg/man/day for the general population (Hunter & Robinson, 1967). Estimates of potential dermal exposure during orchard spraying range from 14.2-15.5 mg/hr, and the potential respiratory exposure was estimated to be 0.03-0.25 mg/hr (Wolfe et al., 1963, 1967).

(b) Air and rain

During an extensive monitoring of the ambient air, dieldrin could be detected in only one out of 9 localities of the US, at a maximum level of 29.7 ng/m^3 (Stanley et al., 1971). In London and suburbs very small quantities (18-21 g/10^{12} g of air) were detected (Abbott et al., 1966), and in airborne dust levels of 0.003 ppm (Cohen & Pinkerton, 1966), 0-8.1 µg/kg (Risebrough et al., 1968) and up to 190 x 10^{-15} g/m^3 of air (Prospero & Seba, 1972) have been found. Average concentrations found in rainwater range from 5-42 ng/l (Abbott et al., 1965; Bevenue et al., 1972; Tarrant & Tatton, 1968; Wheatley & Hardman, 1965).

(c) Soil and water

Dieldrin residue levels in agricultural soils have been the subject of many studies (Deubert & Zuckerman, 1969; Gish, 1970; Saha & Sumner, 1971; Sand et al., 1972; Seal et al., 1967; Trautmann et al., 1968; Wiersma et al., 1972a,b). Different soils exhibit varying degrees of pesticide retention: soil retention is greatest when the organic content is high (Bowman et al., 1965; Winnett & Reed, 1968), and average dieldrin concentrations range from 0.01-16 mg/kg (Sand et al., 1972; Wiersma et al., 1972b). In cranberry bog soil Deubert & Zuckerman (1969) detected an average concentration of 1.18 ppm dieldrin 13 years after its last application. Average concentrations in the soils of 8 cities ranged from <0.01-0.72 mg/kg (Wiersma et al., 1972c).

Application of 0.7 kg dieldrin/acre resulted in average residues of 0.17 ppm in soil and 0.004 ppm in sweet potatoes (Sand et al., 1972). Seal et al. (1967) did not find dieldrin residues in potatoes grown in dieldrin-treated soil, but an average level of 0.05 ppm was found in carrots grown in soil containing an average of 0.19 ppm dieldrin. Wheat seedlings grown in soil containing 12 ppm dieldrin showed an average content of 0.49 ppm (Saha, 1972). Data on residues in potatoes and sugar beets grown in soil with supervised applications of aldrin and dieldrin are summarized in FAO/WHO (1971).

Dieldrin has been found in surface waters, in drinking-water in some locations and in marine life. An average concentration of 0.3 ng/l has been found in drinking-water (Bevenue et al., 1972), and Lenon et al. (1972) found an average of 0.19 µg/l in 50% of cistern water samples taken in one locality in the Virgin Islands.

Many studies on the occurrence of dieldrin in surface waters, mostly rivers and lakes in the US, have been carried out (Breidenbach et al., 1967; Brown & Nishioka, 1967; Herzel, 1972; Johnson & Morris, 1971; Lichtenberg et al., 1970; Manigold & Schulze, 1969); concentrations found ranged from 0-0.1 µg/l.

(d) Animals and plants

Dieldrin is stored in adipose tissue, liver, brain and muscle of mammals, fish and birds, in algae, plankton, insects, earthworms and in the eggs of many bird species.

Fish can build up mg/kg concentrations of dieldrin from ng/l concentrations in water (Reinert, 1970). Hannon et al. (1970) found the following amounts of residues of aldrin + dieldrin: 0.16 ppm in aquatic insects, 0.016 ppm in fish, 0.0007 ppm in plankton and algae and 0.00002 ppm in water. Dieldrin concentrations in fish (including shellfish) from rivers, lakes, estuaries and the sea have also been determined: they are found to be highest in fatty tissues, with concentrations ranging from 0.002-6.7 ppm (Cole et al., 1967; Johnson & Lew, 1970; Stucky, 1970). Residue levels in whole fish ranged from 0-1.59 ppm (Bradshaw et al., 1972; Carr et al., 1972; Henderson et al., 1971; Morris & Johnson, 1971; Reinke et al., 1972) and in shellfish and oysters from 0-0.132 ppm (Bugg et al., 1967; Foehrenbach et al., 1971; Modin, 1969; Rowe et al., 1971).

Dieldrin has also been detected in many bird species (domestic and wild), with average concentrations ranging from 0.01-0.4 ppm in fatty tissue (Greichus et al., 1968; Linder & Dahlgren, 1970; Risebrough et al., 1970) and from 0.6-4.3 ppm in liver (Robinson et al., 1967; Walker et al., 1967), while in the carcass of eagles concentrations from traces to 0.6 ppm have been found (Mulhern et al., 1970; Reichel et al., 1969). Average concentrations in birds' eggs range from 0.01-1.5 ppm (Coulson et al., 1972; Greenberg & Edwards, 1970; Krantz et al., 1970; Vermeer & Reynolds, 1971; Wiemeyer et al., 1972).

(e) Food

In the US, the UK and Japan, a series of analyses of total diets have been reported (Abbott et al., 1969; Corneliussen, 1969, 1970, 1972; Cummings, 1966; Duggan & Corneliussen, 1972; Duggan & Lipscomb, 1969; Duggan & Weatherwax, 1967; Duggan et al., 1966, 1967, 1971; Egan et al., 1966; Martin & Duggan, 1968; McGill & Robinson, 1968; McGill et al., 1969; Robinson & McGill, 1966; Uyeta et al., 1971).

In meat, fish and poultry concentrations of dieldrin found ranged from 0.06 ppm (maximum value) (Corneliussen, 1972; Cummings, 1966) to 0.2 ppm (Corneliussen, 1970; Duggan et al., 1967). Average concentrations in UK mutton fat declined from 1.1 in 1965 to 0.01 ppm in 1970 (Department of Trade & Industry, 1971).

A Joint FAO/WHO Meeting (FAO/WHO, 1971) summarized data from controlled feeding of dieldrin to cattle and poultry: the average ratio of dieldrin levels in fat to levels in feed was 2.43:1 in milking cows and 3.95:1 in steers (Gannon et al., 1959a). Levels of 0.05 ppm dieldrin in rice bran (residues of up to 0.03 ppm are commonly found) resulted in the presence of dieldrin residues in poultry products, up to 0.012 ppm in eggs, 0.20 ppm in fat and 0.02 ppm in poultry meat (FAO/WHO, 1971).

The occurrence of dieldrin in dairy products arises mostly from residues in feed. Many studies on controlled feeding of cows have been carried out, and these are summarized in FAO/WHO (1971) and by Saha (1969). At intake rates of less than 1 ppm, the average ratio of dieldrin levels in milk to levels in feed was about 0.1:1 after 12 weeks (Gannon et al., 1959b; Williams & Mills, 1964). In Denmark, the average concentration in butter fat declined from 0.05 ppm in 1964 to 0.03 ppm in 1966 (Bro-Rasmussen et al., 1968), and that in Great Britain from 0.07 ppm in 1963 to 0.03 ppm in 1964 (Egan et al., 1966). Mean values in butter ranged from <0.01-0.02 ppm in Norway (Bjerk & Sakshaug, 1969), and in the US and Canada average concentrations in milk fat of 0.03-0.04 ppm have been found (Duggan, 1967; Frank et al., 1970).

In total diet studies in the US maximum values ranging from 0.001-0.09 ppm have been found in dairy products (Corneliussen, 1972; Cummings, 1966).

In human milk, 0.001-0.03 ppm have been detected (Curley & Kimbrough, 1969; Egan et al., 1965; Heyndrickx & Maes, 1969; Newton & Greene, 1972).

Many analyses of dieldrin residues in fruits and vegetables have been carried out. In total diet studies only small amounts (maximum values, 0.001-0.03 ppm) have been found (Corneliussen, 1972; Cummings, 1966; Duggan et al., 1967). In grains and cereals maximum values of 0.011-0.014 ppm have been detected, whereas only trace amounts to 0.005 ppm have been detected in oils and fats (Corneliussen, 1969, 1972; Martin & Duggan, 1968), although Addison et al. (1972) found 0.03-0.1 ppm in herring oil.

In the US the total dietary intake was found to range between 0.08-0.05 µg/kg bw/day during the period 1965-1970. This amounts to a 6-year average intake from food of 0.07 µg/kg bw/day (Duggan & Corneliussen, 1972). In the UK for the year 1965 a total intake of 0.30 µg/kg bw/day was calculated (McGill & Robinson, 1968), and a total diet study from 1966-1967 showed the intake of dieldrin to be 0.09 µg/kg bw/day (Abbott et al., 1969). A similar study showed that this had dropped to 0.03 µg/kg bw/day in 1970-1971 (Department of Trade & Industry, 1973). An intake of 0.07 µg/kg bw/day has been estimated in Japan (Uyeta et al., 1971).

No separate acceptable daily intake (ADI) was set by the Joint FAO/WHO Meeting on Pesticide Residues in Food, although a total dieldrin and aldrin ADI of 0-0.0001 mg/kg bw has been recommended (FAO/WHO, 1971).

In the US a threshold limit value of 0.25 mg/m^3 has been established for an 8-hour time-weighted average occupational exposure (US Code of Federal Regulations, 1972).

(f) *Estimation of intake from all sources*

In the US, the UK and Japan the average daily intake of dieldrin from food was reported to have been between 0.03 and 0.34 µg/kg bw/day within the period 1965-1971, intakes being highest in the UK in 1965 (Department of Trade & Industry, 1973; Duggan & Corneliussen, 1972; Duggan & Lipscomb, 1969; Robinson & Roberts, 1969; Uyeta et al., 1971).

Air and water appear to be sources of minor importance; Robinson & Roberts (1969) estimated the intake from drinking-water to be in the order of 0.0003 µg/kg bw/day, and Bevenue et al. (1972) reported an average intake in Hawaii in 1970-1971 of 0.000009 µg/kg bw/day (0.009 ng/kg bw/day).

According to Crabtree (1969), Durham (1969), Hunter et al. (1969), Jansen (1969) and Robinson & Roberts (1969) there is a direct relationship between dieldrin intake and storage in man. They reported storage levels of total dieldrin in body fat in the general population in the years 1961-1968 in the US and UK and 1964-1966 in six other countries ranging from 0.03-0.45 ppm. On the basis of the linear relationship between storage in body fat and exposure (Durham, 1969) and using the above figures, an average intake of dieldrin can be estimated to have ranged from 0.01-0.35 µg/kg bw/day for a 70 kg man; this is in very close agreement with the estimated intake from food given above.

2.3 Analysis

A general approach to the analysis of organochlorine pesticides is given in the preamble (p. 16).

A gel-permeation chromatographic method which requires little or no additional clean-up has been used for the analysis of fish extracts (Stalling et al., 1972). Begliomini & Fravolini (1971) used gas chromatography for the detection of dieldrin in animal feed. An improved gas-liquid chromatographic method for the detection of dieldrin in tobacco has been described by Thimm et al. (1972), and extraction methods for soil (Johnson & Starr, 1972), air (Aue & Teli, 1971) and water (Weil et al., 1972) have also been reported.

Further analytical methods can be found in the references cited in the section on "Occurrence".

3. Biological Data Relevant to the Evaluation of Carcinogenic Risk to Man

3.1 Carcinogenicity and related studies in animals

(a) Oral administration

Mouse: A group of 218 C3HeB/Fe mice, approximately equally divided by sex, was fed a diet containing 10 ppm dieldrin for 2 years, after which all survivors were killed. A similar group of 217 untreated mice was used as controls. Average survival time was 51.4 weeks in treated mice compared with 59.8 weeks in the controls. Liver tumours, diagnosed as hepatic-cell adenomas and described as "extending from very benign lesions to borderline carcinomas", were found in 38 treated and 9 control mice. On average, test mice developed hepatic tumours in 77 weeks and control mice in 89 weeks (Davis & Fitzhugh, 1962). (Evaluation of this study was not possible because of poor survival rate, lack of detailed pathology, loss of information due to the inability to autopsy a large percentage of animals and failure to treat the results in males and females separately.)

A series of experiments on CF1 mice has been reported recently (Thorpe & Walker, 1973; Walker et al., 1973). In all studies, continuous feeding of recrystallized (>99% pure) dieldrin was found to produce liver-cell tumours, while the incidence of tumours at other sites was either unaffected or decreased in relation to the shorter lifespan of animals with liver tumours. Liver-cell tumours were classed as type (a): nodular growths of solid cords of parenchymal cells classified as benign tumours, and type (b): papilliform and adenoid growths with cells proliferating in confluent sheets with necrosis and increased mitoses. Among several hundred mice with liver tumours, metastases were found in 15, all bearing type (b) liver tumours.

In the main experiment, groups of 87-297 mice of each sex were fed diets containing either 0, 0.1, 1.0 or 10 ppm dieldrin for 132 weeks. From the 9th month onwards palpable abdominal masses were detected among mice fed 10 ppm; these mice were killed when the enlargement was considered to be detrimental to their health. Thus, 50% mortality was reached at 15 months among mice fed 10 ppm dieldrin and at 20 months in the other groups.

The incidence of mice with liver tumours (expressed as percentages of the original number of mice) is given in Table 1.

The percentages of liver-tumour-bearing mice in another dose-response study in which exposure to dieldrin lasted 128 weeks are given in Table 2.

In three other groups of 10-24 males and 19-24 females fed 10 ppm dieldrin in different basal diets for 2 years or more, percentages of liver-tumour-bearing mice ranged from 60-86% in males and from 43-63% in females. The percentages of liver-tumour-bearing animals in controls ranged from 23-42% in males and from 11-23% in females.

In a study in which groups of mice were fed 10 ppm dieldrin for different periods and were then allowed to live until 104 weeks, the incidence of liver-cell tumours was recorded (see Table 3) (Walker et al., 1973).

In another study, dieldrin was fed at 10 ppm in the diet for up to 110 weeks to groups of 30 male and 30 female CF1 mice. The incidence of mice with liver-cell tumours was 100% in males and 87% in females, as compared with 24% in 45 male controls and 23% in 44 female controls (Thorpe & Walker, 1973).

Rat: Dieldrin (85% purity) was fed to groups of 40 male and 40 female rats at concentrations of 0, 2.5, 12.5 and 25 ppm in the diet for 2 years. Survival rates were not affected by exposure to dieldrin. Liver pathology only was reported, and no reference was made to the occurrence of tumours (Treon & Cleveland, 1955).

Groups of 12 male and 12 female Osborne-Mendel rats were administered diets containing 0, 0.5, 2, 10, 50, 100 or 150 ppm recrystallized dieldrin (purity ⩾99%) for 2 years. Survival rates were decreased at 50 ppm and above. In groups of rats given 0.5, 2 or 10 ppm dieldrin, the numbers of

Table 1

Dietary concentration (ppm)	No. of animals	% with liver tumours			
		Type a	Type b	Total a + b	(95% fiducial limits)
Males					
0	288	16	4	20	(16-25)
0.1	124	22	4	26	(18-35)
1.0	111	23	8	31	(23-41)
10.0	176	37	57	94	(89-97)
Females					
0	297	13	0	13	(9-17)
0.1	90	23	4	27	(18-38)
1.0	87	31	6	37	(26-48)
10.0	148	37	55	92	(86-96)

Table 2

Dietary concentration (ppm)	No. of animals	% with liver tumours			
		Type a	Type b	Total a + b	(95% fiducial limits)
Males					
0	78	12	0	12	(6-21)
1.25	30	13	7	20	(7-38)
2.5	30	40	3	43	(25-63)
5.0	30	77	10	87	(69-97)
10.0	11	36	9	45	(16-77)
20.0	17	18	53	71	(44-90)
Females					
0	78	10	0	10	(4-19)
1.25	30	17	0	17	(6-35)
2.5	28	39	4	43	(22-63)
5.0	30	43	17	60	(41-77)
10.0	17	41	12	53	(28-77)
20.0	21	24	14	38	(17-62)

Taken from Walker, A.I.T., Thorpe, E. & Stevenson, D.E. (1973) The toxicology of dieldrin (HEOD). I. Long-term oral toxicity studies in mice. Fd Cosmet.Toxicol., 11, 415

Table 3

Duration of feeding (weeks)	No. of animals	No. with liver tumours		
		Type a	Type b	Total a + b
	Males			
0	18	2	0	2
2	13	2	0	2
4	10	0	1	1
8	10	3	1	4
16	11	4	0	4
32	10	4	0	4
64	13	6	7	13
	Females			
0	16	1	0	1
2	9	2	0	2
4	12	3	1	4
8	12	4	0	4
16	8	3	0	3
32	10	4	0	4
64	9	6	2	8

Taken from Walker, A.I.T., Thorpe, E. & Stevenson, D.E. (1973) The toxicology of dieldrin (HEOD). I. Long-term oral toxicity studies in mice. Fd Cosmet. Toxicol., 11, 415

tumour-bearing animals were 8/22, 8/23 and 4/18 at 0.5, 2 and 10 ppm, respectively, compared to 3/17 in the controls. These groups showed a survival rate of 75% at 18 months, which was comparable to that in the controls. Among treated rats there were 9 lymphomas (1 in the controls), 5 benign and 2 malignant mammary tumours (1 benign tumour in the controls) and 6 tumours at other sites (1 in the controls) (Fitzhugh et al., 1964).

(These results were considered by the authors as evidence of "some general type of effect that increased tumour production, without causing any single type of tumour to predominate". However, the difference between 20/63 tumour-bearing rats in the treated groups and 3/17 in the controls is not significant (χ^2 = 0.71, P>0.05).)

Groups of 25 male and 25 female CFE rats were administered diets containing 0.1, 1.0 or 10 ppm recrystallized dieldrin (purity 99%) for 2 years. A group of 45 males and 45 females received the control diet. At the end of the 2-year period the mortality was 58% in male and 58% in female controls and ranged from 35-61% in the treated groups, being highest at the 10 ppm level. The number of tumour-bearing animals was 28% in control males and ranged from 22-35% in the treated males, with no dose-response trend. Among the females there were 44% bearing tumours in controls and 52-65% in treated animals. The incidences of thyroid, pituitary, mammary and other tumours were comparable in all groups. Microscopic hyperplastic liver nodules were found in 1 control female and in 3 females receiving 10 ppm dieldrin (Walker et al., 1969).

Groups of 50 male and 50 female Osborne-Mendel rats were administered diets containing 20, 30 or 50 ppm dieldrin (technical, 100% active ingredient) and were compared to a control group of 100 rats of each sex. Survival rate was not affected in males, while in females the mean survival times were 19.5 months in the controls, 20.5 months in those fed 20 ppm, 17.4 months with 30 ppm and 16.6 months with 50 ppm. The proportion of tumour-bearing rats and the incidence of mammary tumours, lymphomas and other tumours in treated rats were similar to those observed in control animals. No liver-cell tumours were reported (Deichmann et al., 1970).

Dog: Groups of 5 dogs of each sex were given oral doses of 0, 0.005 and 0.05 mg/kg bw dieldrin by capsule daily for 2 years and then killed. Liver:body weight ratios were increased in dogs given 0.05 mg/kg bw/day dieldrin. No tumours were found (Walker et al., 1969). (The duration of this study was too short for it to be evaluated.)

Monkey: In an experiment reported as in progress, 31 rhesus monkeys were fed dieldrin in concentrations of 0.01, 0.1, 0.5, 1.0 or 5.0 ppm in the diet for 3 years. No excess of tumours was observed throughout this period (Zavon et al., 1967). (The duration of the study was too short for it to be evaluated.)

3.2 Other relevant biological data

(a) Metabolism and storage in animals

When ^{14}C-dieldrin was administered to rats and mice as a single dose by gavage, 10 times as much radioactivity was found in faeces compared to urine in both species. Approximately 50-70% of the radioactivity was eliminated within 1 week. Of the total daily radioactivity found in the urine, the amount of dieldrin excreted by rats varied from 2-22%; in addition, "pentachloroketone" (1)* was identified in rat urine, its proportion increasing from 3 to 67% over the 8 days after administration. These two compounds were not detected in mouse urine (Baldwin et al., 1972).

In rat faeces within the first 24 hours after dosing, 36% of the radioactivity was identified as dieldrin; this rapidly decreased to undetectable levels within the next 4 days. In mouse faeces, the amount of radioactivity identified as dieldrin was 22% on the first day and 14.5% on the 6th day. Both the mouse and the rat excreted high levels of a 9-hydroxy dieldrin (2)* in faeces (46% and 26%, respectively), and about one third of the dieldrin was excreted by the two species as unidentified metabolites. One of the faecal metabolites in the rat was identified as 6,7-trans-dihydroaldrindiol (3)*, and one of the urinary metabolites as hexachlorohexahydromethanoindene-1,3-dicarboxylic acid (4)* (Baldwin et al., 1972). For

---

* For structure see page 141.

further details on identified mammalian metabolites see Brooks (1969) and Menzie (1969).

In rats fed 50 ppm in the diet, the concentration of dieldrin increased for the first 9 days in liver and blood and then remained fairly constant for the next 6 months. Equilibrium was reached in adipose tissue in 16 days. The mean ratios for levels in blood, liver and adipose tissue after equilibrium was reached were approximately 1:30:500 (Deichmann et al., 1968).

Rats were given 75 ppm dieldrin in the diet for 12 months, and within 15 days after cessation of exposure the concentration of dieldrin in adipose tissue had dropped to half of the concentration found after 12 months' exposure (Robinson & Roberts, 1968).

Walker et al. (1971) reported that the photoisomerisation product of dieldrin (see section 1.3 (e)) was stored at a higher rate in the tissues of female rats than in those of males, but that this was not true for dogs.

Transplacental passage of dieldrin has been demonstrated in rabbits (Hathway et al., 1967), in rats (Eliason & Posner, 1971), in pigs (Uzoukwu & Sleight, 1972) and in cows (Braund et al., 1967).

(b) Metabolism and storage in man

Richardson & Robinson (1971) reported that workers with occupational exposure to dieldrin and aldrin excreted 9-hydroxy-dieldrin (2)[*] in the faeces. Concentrations of dieldrin in the plasma of small groups of pregnant women ranged from 0.0001-0.0061 ppm (Curley & Kimbrough, 1969), and the concentration in whole-cord blood of newborn babies ranged from 0.0002-0.0015 ppm (Curley et al., 1969). Similar blood levels in mothers and newborn babies were also reported by Radomski et al. (1971).

Low concentrations of dieldrin have been found in human milk: in Australia, it was found in 29/67 milk samples, at concentrations ranging from 0.001-0.029 ppm (Newton & Greene, 1972); in the US, Curley & Kimbrough (1969) found dieldrin concentrations ranging from 0.0029-0.0146 ppm, and

---

[*] For structure see page 141.

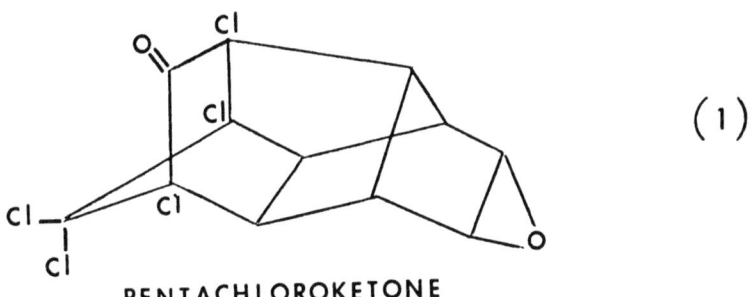

PENTACHLOROKETONE (1)

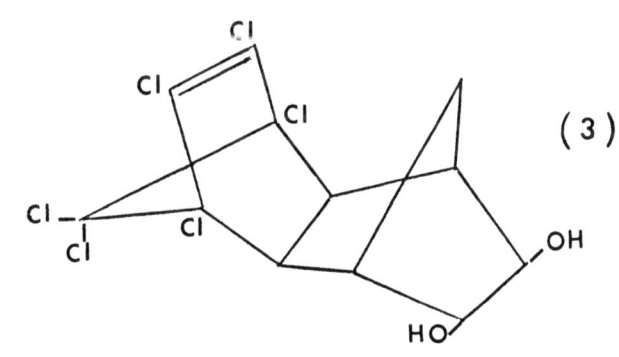

9-HYDROXYDIELDRIN (2)

6,7-TRANS-DIHYDROALDRINDIOL (3)

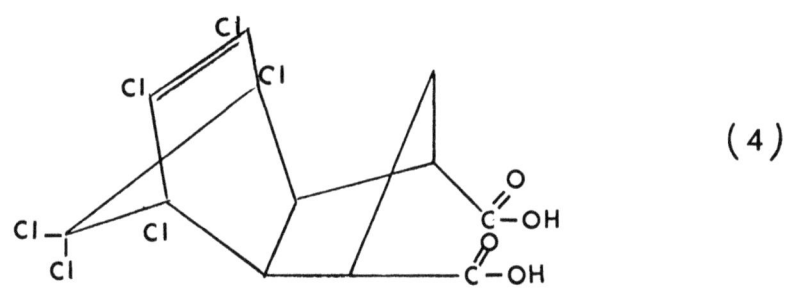

HEXACHLOROHEXAHYDROMETHANOINDENE-
1,3-DICARBOXYLIC ACID (4)

Dyment et al. (1971) reported similar concentrations, with a mean of 0.0033 ppm. Tuinstra (1971) summarized the different dieldrin concentrations in human milk reported from various countries: the mean concentration found in The Netherlands was 0.003 ppm, and in Belgium 0.0035 ppm.

Acute dieldrin poisoning in two children resulted in the death of one child. Three days after ingestion, the concentration of dieldrin in the serum in the non-fatal poisoning was 0.27 ppm, and this decreased to 0.11 ppm within 2 weeks. A fat specimen obtained 3 days after ingestion contained 47 ppm dieldrin; six months later the amount in adipose tissue had dropped to about 15 ppm, and after 8 months it was still at the same level (Garrettson & Curley, 1969).

Hunter & Robinson (1967) gave small doses of dieldrin to human volunteers. A daily ingestion of 50 µg/day resulted at the end of 18 months in a body burden 4 times higher than that of the general population; and when 211 µg/day were ingested for a period of 18 months the body burden was 10 times higher than that of the general population.

Workers exposed occupationally to dieldrin and aldrin had a mean concentration of 0.0185 ppm dieldrin in plasma and stored a mean of 5.67 ppm in adipose tissue. None of these workers showed any ill effects (Hayes & Curley, 1968). The dieldrin concentrations in adipose tissue of the general population between 1961 and 1964 ranged from 0.04 ppm in India to 0.31 ppm in the US (Durham, 1969). Abbott et al. (1972) reported an arithmetic mean concentration of dieldrin in adipose tissue of the general population in the UK of 0.16 ppm for the period of 1969-1971. Curley et al. (1973) reported average levels of 0.13 ppm dieldrin in Japanese adipose tissue samples in the general population in 1971.

For additional data see table in appendix p. 224.

3.3 Observations in man

(a) Studies on workers exposed to dieldrin

A study was undertaken in 1968 on 233 workers employed in a factory which had been manufacturing aldrin and dieldrin since 1954-1955, endrin since 1957 and telodrin during 1958-1965. Lengths of exposure ranged from 4-13.3 years (average, 7.6 years). One hundred and eighty-one workers were still employed by the same firm at the time of the study, and their average age was 41 years (range, 22-64). Only 2 deaths had occurred, and one had been caused by stomach cancer (Jager, 1970). The 52 workers who had left the company have been the subject of a subsequent report. Average age at the time of this survey was 47.4 years (range, 29-72), average occupational exposure was 6.6 years (4.0-12.3) and average time since the end of exposure was 7.4 years (4.5-16). Only one death was recorded, and this had not been caused by cancer (Versteeg & Jager, 1973).

(b) Concentration of dieldrin in tissues of terminal patients

In a study on 38 persons dying between the ages of 36-88 years, it was found that among 19 patients with lower tissue levels of organochlorine (total DDT + dieldrin + heptachlor epoxide), 4 had malignant tumours, whereas the corresponding figure for the 19 patients with higher levels was 9 (Casarett et al., 1968).

In another investigation of various pesticides in fat samples, the average concentration (in ppm) of dieldrin was 0.55 ± 0.34 in 40 cases of carcinoma, 0.47 ± 0.22 in 5 cases of leukaemia, 0.51 ± 0.18 in 5 cases of Hodgkin's disease and 0.21 ± 0.15 in 42 "control" cases (Radomski et al., 1968).

4. Comments on Data Reported and Evaluation[1]

4.1 Animal data

Dieldrin was tested by the oral route only in mice and rats. The hepatocarcinogenicity of dieldrin in the mouse has been demonstrated and confirmed in several experiments, and some of the liver-cell tumours were found to metastasize. A dose-response effect has been demonstrated in both sexes with an increased tumour incidence in females at the lowest dose

---

[1] See also the section "Animal Data in Relation to the Evaluation of Risk to Man" in the introduction to this volume.

tested, 0.1 ppm in the diet (corresponding to about 0.015 mg/kg bw/day). In mice, there is no evidence of carcinogenicity in organs other than the liver.

The available data in rats have not provided evidence of carcinogenicity at levels of up to 50 ppm in the diet (corresponding to an intake of about 2.5 mg/kg bw/day).

The experiments in dogs and monkeys were too limited in duration and/or group sizes to allow any conclusions to be made.

4.2 Human data

The epidemiological study carried out on occupationally exposed workers does not allow any conclusions to be made concerning the existence of an excess risk of developing cancer.

Although fat concentrations of dieldrin residues were higher in terminal cancer patients than in control patients, this finding is inconclusive as to a causal relationship.

5. References

Abbott, D.C., Harrison, R.B., Tatton, J.O'G. & Thomson, J. (1965) Organochlorine pesticides in the atmospheric environment. Nature (Lond.), 208, 1317

Abbott, D.C., Harrison, R.B., Tatton, J.O'G. & Thomson, J. (1966) Organochlorine pesticides in the atmosphere. Nature (Lond.), 211, 259

Abbott, D.C., Holmes, D.C. & Tatton, J.O'G. (1969) Pesticide residues in the total diet in England and Wales 1966-67. II. Organochlorine pesticide residues in the total diet. J. Sci. Fd Agric., 20, 245

Abbott, D.C., Collins, G.B. & Goulding, R. (1972) Organochlorine pesticide residues in human fat in the United Kingdom, 1969-1971. Brit. med. J., ii, 553

Addison, R.F., Zinck, M.E. & Ackman, R.G. (1972) Residues of organochlorine pesticides and polychlorinated biphenyls in some commercially produced Canadian marine oils. J. Fish. Res. Board Canada, 29, 349

Anon. (1972a) Chemical Marketing Reporter, November 27, pp. 3, 18

Anon. (1972b) Le DDT interdit en Suisse depuis le 1er avril 1972. Phytoma, 239, 37 (An English abstract is given in Health Aspects of Pesticides Abstract Bulletin, 72-2520)

Aue, W.A. & Teli, P.M. (1971) Sampling of air pollutants with support-bonded chromatographic phases. J. Chromat., 62, 15

Baldwin, M.K., Robinson, J. & Parke, D.V. (1972) A comparison of the metabolism of HEOD (dieldrin) in the CF1 mouse with that in the CFE rat. Fd Cosmet. Toxicol., 10, 333

Begliomini, A. & Fravolini, A. (1971) Residui di insetticidi nei mangimi. II. Identificazione e dosaggio gas cromatografico di insetticidi clorurati ed esteri fosforici in mangimi composti. Arch. vet. ital., 22, 109

Bevenue, A., Hylin, J.W., Kawano, Y. & Kelley, T.W. (1972) Organochlorine pesticide residues in water, sediment, algae and fish, Hawaii, 1970-71. Pest. Monit. J., 6, 56

Bjerk, J.E. & Sakshaug, J. (1969) Residues of organochlorine insecticides in samples of Norwegian butter, 1968. Nord. vet. Med., 21, 635

Bowman, M.C., Schechter, M.S. & Carter, R.L. (1965) Behaviour of chlorinated insecticides in a broad spectrum of soil types. J. agric. Fd Chem., 13, 360

Bradshaw, J.S., Loveridge, E.L., Rippee, K.P., Peterson, J.L., White, D.A., Barton, J.R. & Fuhriman, D.K. (1972) Seasonal variations in residues of chlorinated hydrocarbon pesticides in the water of the Utah Lake drainage system - 1970 and 1971. Pest. Monit. J., 6, 166

Braund, D.G., Brown, L.D., Leeling, N.C., Zabik, M.J. & Hubert, J.T. (1967) Storage, excretion and placental transfer of dieldrin by dairy heifers contaminated during three stages of gestation. J. Dairy Sci., 50, 991

Breidenbach, A.W., Gunnerson, C.G., Kawahara, F.K., Lichtenberg, J.J. & Green, R.S. (1967) Chlorinated hydrocarbon pesticides in major river basins, 1957-1965. Publ. Hlth Rep., 82, 139

Brooks, G.T. (1969) The metabolism of diene-organochlorine (cyclodiene) insecticides. Res. Rev., 27, 81

Bro-Rasmussen, F., Dalgaard-Mikkelsen, Sv., Jakobson, Th., Koch, Sv.O., Rodin, F., Uhl, E. & Voldum-Clausen, K. (1968) Examinations of Danish milk and butter for contaminating organochlorine insecticides. Res. Rev., 23, 55

Brown, E. & Nishioka, Y.A. (1967) Pesticides in selected western streams - a contribution to the national program. Pest. Monit. J., 1, ii, 38

Bugg, J.C., Jr, Higgins, J.E. & Robertson, E.A., Jr (1967) Chlorinated pesticide levels in the eastern oyster (Crassostrea virginica) from selected areas of the South Atlantic and Gulf of Mexico. Pest. Monit. J., 1, iii, 9

California Department of Agriculture (1972) Pesticide Use Report, 1971, Sacramento, pp. 62-63

California Department of Agriculture (1973) Pesticide Use Report, 1972, Sacramento, pp. 67-68

Carr, R.L., Finsterwalder, C.E. & Schibi, M.J. (1972) Chemical residues in Lake Erie fish, 1970-71. Pest. Monit. J., 6, 23

Casarett, L.J., Fuyer, G.C., Yauger, W.L., Jr & Klemmer, H.W. (1968) Organochlorine pesticide residues in human tissue - Hawaii. Arch. environm. Hlth, 17, 306

Chemical Information Services, Ltd. (1973) Directory of West European Chemical Producers, Oceanside, NY

Cohen, J.M. & Pinkerton, C. (1966) Widespread translocation of pesticides by air transport and rainout. Organic Pesticides in the Environment, Adv. Chem. Ser., 60, 163

Cole, H., Bradford, A., Barry, D., Baumgarner, P. & Frear, D.E.H. (1967) Pesticides in hatchery trout - differences between species and residue levels occurring in commercial fish food. Pest. Monit. J., 1, ii, 35

Corneliussen, P.E. (1969) Pesticide residues in total diet samples (IV). Pest. Monit. J., 2, 140

Corneliussen, P.E. (1970) Pesticide residues in total diet samples (V). Pest. Monit. J., 4, 89

Corneliussen, P.E. (1972) Pesticide residues in total diet samples (VI). Pest. Monit. J., 5, 313

Coulson, J.C., Deans, I.R., Potts, G.R., Robinson, J. & Crabtree, A.N. (1972) Changes in organochlorine contamination of the marine environment of eastern Britain monitored by shag eggs. Nature (Lond.), 236, 454

Crabtree, A.M. (1969) The concentration of organochlorine insecticides in human fat and blood from Australia. Tunstall Laboratory Report No. TL GR 0059-69, Sittingbourne, Kent, Shell Research Ltd.

Cummings, J.G. (1966) Pesticides in the total diet. Res. Rev., 16, 30

Curley, A. & Kimbrough, R. (1969) Chlorinated hydrocarbon insecticides in plasma and milk of pregnant and lactating women. Arch. environm. Hlth, 18, 156

Curley, A., Copeland, M.F. & Kimbrough, R.D. (1969) Chlorinated hydrocarbon insecticides in organs of stillborn and blood of newborn babies. Arch. environm. Hlth, 19, 628

Curley, A., Burse, V.W., Jennings, R.W., Villanueva, E.C., Tomatis, L. & Akazaki, K. (1973) Chlorinated hydrocarbon pesticides and related compounds in adipose tissue from people of Japan. Nature (Lond.), 242, 338

Davis, K.J. & Fitzhugh, O.G. (1962) Tumorigenic potential of aldrin and dieldrin for mice. Toxicol. appl. Pharmacol., 4, 187

Deichmann, W.B., Dressler, I., Keplinger, M. & MacDonald, W.E. (1968) Retention of dieldrin in blood, liver and fat of rats fed dieldrin for six months. Industr. Med. Surg., 37, 837

Deichmann, W.B., MacDonald, W.E., Blum, E., Bevilacqua, M., Radomski, J., Keplinger, M. & Balkus, M. (1970) Tumorigenicity of aldrin, dieldrin and endrin in the albino rat. Industr. Med. Surg., 39, 426

Department of Trade & Industry (1971) Report of the Government Chemist 1970, London, HMSO

Department of Trade & Industry (1973) Report of the Government Chemist 1972 (in press)

Deubert, K.H. & Zuckerman, B.M. (1969) Distribution of dieldrin and DDT in cranberry bog soil. Pest. Monit. J., 2, 172

Duggan, R.E. (1967) Chlorinated pesticide residues in fluid milk and other dairy products in the United States. Pest. Monit. J., 1, iii, 2

Duggan, R.E. & Corneliussen, P.E. (1972) Dietary intake of pesticide chemicals in the United States (III), June 1968-April 1970. Pest. Monit. J., 5, 331

Duggan, R.E. & Lipscomb, G.Q. (1969) Dietary intake of pesticide chemicals in the United States (II), June 1966-April 1968. Pest. Monit. J., 2, 153

Duggan, R.E. & Weatherwax, J.R. (1967) Dietary intake of pesticide chemicals. Science, 157, 1006

Duggan, R.E., Barry, H.C. & Johnson, L.Y. (1966) Pesticide residues in total diet samples. Science, 151, 101

Duggan, R.E., Barry, H.C. & Johnson, L.Y. (1967) Pesticide residues in total diet samples (II). Pest. Monit. J., 1, ii, 2

Duggan, R.E., Lipscomb, G.Q., Cox, E.L., Heatwole, R.E. & Kling, R.C. (1971) Pesticide residue levels in foods in the United States from July 1, 1963 to June 30, 1969. Pest. Monit. J., 5, 73

Durham, W.F. (1969) Body burden of pesticides in man. Ann. N.Y. Acad. Sci., 160, 183

Dyment, P.G., Hebertson, L.M., Decker, W.J., Gomes, E.D. & Wiseman, J.S. (1971) Relationship between levels of chlorinated hydrocarbon insecticides in human milk and serum. Bull. environm. Contam. Toxicol., 6, 449

Economic Documantation Office (1973) Entoma Europe, 1973-75, Hilversum, The Netherlands, pp. 103-106

Egan, H., Goulding, R., Roburn, J. & Tatton, J.O'G. (1965) Organochlorine pesticide residues in human fat and human milk. Brit. med. J., iii, 66

Egan, H., Holmes, D.C., Roburn, J. & Tatton, J.O'G. (1966) Pesticide residues in foodstuffs in Great Britain. II. Persistent organochlorine pesticide residues in selected foods. J. Sci. Fd Agric., 17, 563

Eliason, B.C. & Posner, H.S. (1971) Placental passage of ^{14}C-dieldrin altered by gestational age and plasma proteins. Amer. J. Obstet. Gynec., 111, 925

FAO (1972) FAO Production Yearbook - 1971, 25, Rome, p. 505

FAO/WHO (1967) Evaluation of some pesticide residues in food. FAO/PL: CP/15; WHO/Food Add./67.32

FAO/WHO (1968) 1967 Evaluation of some pesticide residues in food. FAO/PL: 1967/M/11/1; WHO/Food Add./68.30

FAO/WHO (1969) 1968 Evaluations of some pesticide residues in food. FAO/PL/1968/M/9/1; WHO/Food Add./69.35

FAO/WHO (1970) 1969 Evaluations of some pesticide residues in food. FAO/PL/1969/M/17/1; WHO/Food Add./70.38

FAO/WHO (1971) 1970 Evaluation of some pesticide residues in food. FAO/AGP/1970/M/12/1; WHO/Food Add./71.42, p. 210

FAO/WHO (1973) Pesticide residues in food. Report of the 1972 Joint FAO/WHO Meeting. Wld Hlth Org. techn. Rep. Ser., No. 525, p. 31

Fitzhugh, O.G., Nelson, A.A. & Quaife, M.L. (1964) Chronic oral toxicity of aldrin and dieldrin in rats and dogs. Fd Cosmet. Toxicol., 2, 551

Foehrenbach, J., Mahmood, G. & Sullivan, D. (1971) Chlorinated hydrocarbon residues in shellfish (Pelecypoda) from estuaries of Long Island, New York. Pest. Monit. J., 5, 242

Frank, R., Braun, H.E. & McWade, J.W. (1970) Chlorinated hydrocarbon residues in the milk supply of Ontario, Canada. Pest. Monit. J., 4, 31

Frear, D.E.H., ed. (1972) Pesticide Handbook - Entoma, 24th ed., State College, Pennsylvania, College Science Publishers, p. 118

Galley, R.A.E. (1970) Chlorkohlenwasserstoffe: 4. Cyclodien-Insektizide. In: Wegler, R., ed., Chemie der Pflanzenschutz und Schädlings-bekämpfungsmittel, Berlin, Heidelberg, New York, Springer-Verlag, 1, pp. 163-192 (in English)

Gannon, N., Link, R.P. & Decker, G.C. (1959a) Pesticide residues in meat. Storage of dieldrin in tissues of steers, hogs, lambs and poultry fed dieldrin in their diets. J. agric. Fd Chem., 7, 826

Gannon, N., Link, R.P. & Decker, G.C. (1959b) Pesticide residues in meat and milk. Storage of dieldrin in tissues and its excretion in milk of dairy cows fed dieldrin in their diets. J. agric. Fd Chem., 7, 824

Garrettson, L.K. & Curley, A. (1969) Dieldrin. Studies in a poisoned child. Arch. environm. Hlth, 19, 814

Gish, C.D. (1970) Organochlorine insecticide residues in soils and soil invertebrates from agricultural lands. Pest. Monit. J., 3, 241

Greenberg, R.E. & Edwards, W.R. (1970) Insecticide residue levels in eggs of wild pheasants in Illinois. Trans. Ill. State Acad. Sci., 63, 136

Greichus, Y.A., Greichus, A. & Reider, E.G. (1968) Insecticide residues in grouse and pheasant of South Dakota. Pest. Monit. J., 2, 90

Hannon, M.R., Greichus, Y.A., Applegate, R.L. & Fox, A.C. (1970) Ecological distribution of pesticides in Lake Poinsett, South Dakota. Trans. amer. Fish. Soc., 99, 496

Hathway, D.E., Moss, J.A., Rose, J.A. & Williams, D.J.M. (1967) Transport of dieldrin from mother to blastocyst and from mother to foetus in pregnant rabbits. Europ. J. Pharmacol., 1, 167

Hayashi, M. (1971) Residues of agricultural drugs and health of children. Shohni Hoken Kenkyu (Children Hlth Study), 30, 1

Hayes, W.J. & Curley, A. (1968) Storage and excretion of dieldrin and related compounds. Effect of occupational exposure. Arch. environm. Hlth, 16, 155

Henderson, C., Inglis, A. & Johnson, W.L. (1971) Organochlorine insecticide residues in fish - fall 1969, national pesticide monitoring program. Pest. Monit. J., 5, 1

Herzel, F. (1972) Organochlorine insecticides in surface waters in Germany - 1970 and 1971. Pest. Monit. J., 6, 179

Heyndrickx, A. & Maes, R. (1969) The excretion of chlorinated hydrocarbon insecticides in human mother milk. J. Pharm. belg., 24, 459

Hunter, C.G. & Robinson, J. (1967) Pharmacodynamics of dieldrin (HEOD). I. Ingestion by human subjects for 18 months. Arch. environm. Hlth, 15, 614

Hunter, C.G., Robinson, J. & Roberts, M. (1969) Pharmacodynamics of dieldrin (HEOD). Ingestion by human subjects for 18 to 24 months and post-exposure for eight months. Arch. environm. Hlth, 18, 12

Jager, K.W. (1970) Aldrin, dieldrin, endrin and telodrin. An epidemiological and toxicological study of long-term occupational exposure. Amsterdam, London, New York, Elsevier, pp. 60, 121-131

Jansen, J.D. (1969) Letter to A.M. Coetzee dated 25 July 1969. Cited in: 1970 Evaluations of some pesticide residues in food. WHO/Food Add./71.42, p. 196

Japan Chemical Week, ed. (1973) Japan Chemical Directory, Osaka, The Chemical Daily Co., Ltd., p. 357

Johnson, D.W. & Lew, S. (1970) Chlorinated hydrocarbon pesticides in representative fishes of Southern Arizona. Pest. Monit. J., 4, 57

Johnson, L.G. & Morris, R.L. (1971) Chlorinated hydrocarbon pesticides in Iowa rivers. Pest. Monit. J., 4, 216

Johnson, O. (1972) Pesticides '72. Chemical Week, June 21, p. 57

Johnson, R.E. & Starr, R.I. (1972) Ultrarapid extraction of insecticides from soil using a new ultrasonic technique. J. agric. Fd Chem., 20, 48

Krantz, W.C., Mulhern, B.M., Bagley, G.E., Sprunt, A., IV, Ligas, F.J. & Robertson, W.B., Jr (1970) Organochlorine and heavy metal residues in bald eagle eggs. Pest. Monit. J., 4, 136

Lenon, H., Curry, L., Miller, A. & Patulski, D. (1972) Insecticide residues in water and sediment from cisterns on the US and British Virgin Islands. Pest. Monit. J., 6, 188

Lichtenberg, J.J., Eichelberger, J.W., Dressman, R.C. & Longbottom, J.E. (1970) Pesticides in surface waters of the United States - a 5-year summary, 1964-68. Pest. Monit. J., 4, 71

Linder, R.L. & Dahlgren, R.B. (1970) Occurrence of organochlorine insecticides in pheasants of South Dakota. Pest. Monit. J., 3, 227

Lipson, M. (1970) Wool. Insectproofing. In: Kirk, R.E. & Othmer, D.F., eds., Encyclopedia of Chemical Technology, 2nd ed., New York, John Wiley & Sons, Vol. 22, p. 406

Manigold, D.B. & Schulze, J.A. (1969) Pesticides in selected western streams - a progress report. Pest. Monit. J., 3, 124

Martin, R.J. & Duggan, R.E. (1968) Pesticide residues in total diet samples (III). Pest. Monit. J., 1, iv, 11

McGill, A.E.J. & Robinson, J. (1968) Organochlorine insecticide residues in complete prepared meals: a 12-month survey in SE England. Fd Cosmet. Toxicol., 6, 45

McGill, A.E.J., Robinson, J. & Stein, M. (1969) Residues of dieldrin (HEOD) in complete prepared meals in Great Britain during 1967. Nature (Lond.), 221, 761

Menzie, C.M. (1969) Aldrin, dieldrin, isodrin, endrin. In: Metabolism of Pesticides, Bureau of Sports Fisheries and Wildlife, Special Scientific Report - Wildlife, No. 127, Washington DC, US Department of the Interior, p. 24

Modin, J.C. (1969) Chlorinated hydrocarbon pesticides in California bays and estuaries. Pest. Monit. J., 3, 1

Morris, R.L. & Johnson, L.G. (1971) Dieldrin levels in fish from Iowa streams. Pest. Monit. J., 5, 12

Mulhern, B.M., Reichel, W.L., Locke, L.N., Lamont, T.G., Belisle, A., Cromartie, E., Bagley, G.E. & Prouty, R.M. (1970) Organochlorine residues and autopsy data from bald eagles, 1966-68. Pest. Monit. J., 4, 141

Newton, K.G. & Greene, N.C. (1972) Organochlorine pesticide residue levels in human milk - Victoria, Australia, 1970. Pest. Monit. J., 6, 4

Ogata, I. (1972) Merits and demerits of DDT from the viewpoint of sanitation. Gekkan Yakuji (Pharm. Monit.), 14, 1788 (An English abstract is given in Health Aspects of Pesticides Abstract Bulletin, No. 73-0013)

Prospero, J.M. & Seba, D.B. (1972) Some additional measurements of pesticides in the lower atmosphere of the northern equatorial Atlantic Ocean. Atmos. Environm., 6, 363

Radomski, J.L., Deichmann, W.B. & Clizer, E.E. (1968) Pesticide concentrations in the liver, brain and adipose tissue of terminal hospital patients. Fd Cosmet. Toxicol., 6, 209

Radomski, J.L., Astolfi, E., Deichmann, W.B. & Rey, A.A. (1971) Blood levels of organochlorine pesticides in Argentina's occupationally and non-occupationally exposed adults, children and newborn infants. Toxicol. appl. Pharmacol., 20, 186

Ragno, M., ed. (1972) Repertorio Chimico Italiano, Industriale e Commerciale, Milano, Asiminum

Reichel, W.L., Cromartie, E., Lamont, T.G., Mulhern, B.M. & Prouty, R.M. (1969) Pesticide residues in eagles. Pest. Monit. J., 3, 142

Reinert, R.E. (1970) Pesticide concentrations in Great Lakes fish. Pest. Monit. J., 3, 233

Reinke, J., Uthe, J.F. & Jamieson, D. (1972) Organochlorine pesticide residues in commercially caught fish in Canada, 1970. Pest. Monit. J., 6, 43

Richardson, A. & Robinson, J. (1971) The identification of a major metabolite of HEOD (dieldrin) in human faeces. Xenobiotica, 1, 213

Risebrough, R.W., Huggett, R.J., Griffin, J.J. & Goldgerg, E.D. (1968) Pesticides: transatlantic movements in the northeast trades. Science, 159, 1233

Risebrough, R.W., Florant, G.L. & Berger, D.D. (1970) Organochlorine pollutants in peregrines and merlins migrating through Wisconsin. Can. Fld-Natur., 84, 247

Robinson, J. & McGill, A.E.J. (1966) Organochlorine insecticide residues in complete prepared meals in Great Britain during 1965. Nature (Lond.), 212, 1037

Robinson, J. & Roberts, M. (1968) Accumulation, distribution and elimination of organochlorine insecticides by vertebrates. In: Symposium on Physicochemical and Biophysical Factors Affecting the Activity of Pesticides, London, 1967, London, Society of Chemical Industry, pp. 106-119

Robinson, J. & Roberts, M. (1969) Estimation of the exposure of the general population to dieldrin (HEOD). Fd Cosmet. Toxicol., 7, 501

Robinson, J., Richardson, A. & Bush, B. (1966) A photoisomerization product of dieldrin. Bull. environm. Contam. Toxicol., 1, 127

Robinson, J., Richardson, A., Crabtree, A.N., Coulson, J.C. & Potts, G.R. (1967) Organochlorine residues in marine organisms. Nature (Lond.), 214, 1307

Rosen, J.D., Sutherland, D.J. & Lipton, G.R. (1966) The photochemical isomerization of dieldrin and endrin and effects on toxicity. Bull. environm. Contam. Toxicol., 1, 133

Rowe, D.R., Canter, L.W., Snyder, P.J. & Mason, J.W. (1971) Dieldrin and endrin concentrations in a Louisiana estuary. Pest. Monit. J., 4, 177

Saha, J.G. (1969) Significance of organochlorine residues in fresh plants as possible contaminants of milk and beef products. Res. Rev., 26, 89

Saha, J.G. (1972) Residues in seedlings of ten wheat varieties grown in dieldrin-treated soil. J. econ. Entomol., 65, 302

Saha, J.G. & Sumner, A.K. (1971) Organochlorine insecticide residues in soil from vegetable farms in Saskatchewan. Pest. Monit. J., 5, 28

Sand, P.F., Wiersma, G.B. & Landry, J.L. (1972) Pesticide residues in sweet potatoes and soil - 1969. Pest. Monit. J., 5, 342

Seal, W.L., Dawsey, L.H. & Cavin, G.E. (1967) Monitoring for chlorinated hydrocarbon pesticides in soil and root crops in the eastern states in 1965. Pest. Monit. J., 1, iii, 22

Stalling, D.L., Tindle, R.C. & Johnson, J.L. (1972) Clean-up of pesticide and polychlorinated biphenyl residues in fish extracts by gel-permeation chromatography. J. Ass. off. analyt. Chem., 55, 32

Stanley, C.W., Barney, J.E., II, Helton, M.R. & Yobs, A.R. (1971) Measurement of atmospheric levels of pesticides. Environm. Sci. Technol., 5, 430

Stucky, N.P. (1970) Pesticide residues in channel catfish from Nebraska. Pest. Monit. J., 4, 62

Tarrant, K.R. & Tatton, J.O'G. (1968) Organochlorine pesticides in rainwater in the British Isles. Nature (Lond.), 219, 725

Thimm, H.F., Belcher, R.S. & Briner, G.P. (1972) Estimation of dieldrin in cured tobacco. Pest. Sci., 3, 175

Thorpe, E. & Walker, A.I.T. (1973) The toxicology of dieldrin (HEOD). II. Comparative long-term oral toxicity studies in mice with dieldrin, DDT, phenobarbitone, β-BHC and γ-BHC. Fd Cosmet. Toxicol., 11, 433

Trautmann, W.L., Chesters, G. & Pionke, H.B. (1968) Organochlorine insecticide composition of randomly selected soils from nine states - 1967. Pest. Monit. J., 2, 93

Treon, J.F. & Cleveland, F.P. (1955) Toxicity of certain chlorinated hydrocarbon insecticides for laboratory animals with special reference to aldrin and dieldrin. J. agric. Fd Chem., 3, 402

Tuinstra, L.G.M.Th. (1971) Organochlorine insecticide residues in human milk in the Leiden region. Neth. Milk Dairy J., 25, 24

US Code of Federal Regulations (1972) Washington DC, US Government Printing Office, 29 CFR 1910.93

US Environmental Protection Agency (1973a) Environmental News, August 3, Washington DC, US Government Printing Office

US Environmental Protection Agency (1973b) EPA Compendium of Registered Pesticides, Washington DC, US Government Printing Office, pp. III-D-24.1 - III-D-24.11

US Environmental Protection Agency (1973c) Water pollution prevention and control. Proposed list of toxic pollutants. US Federal Register, 38, No. 129, Washington DC, US Government Printing Office, pp. 18044-18045

US Tariff Commission (1951) Synthetic Organic Chemicals, United States Production and Sales, 1950 Second Series, Report No. 173, Washington DC, US Government Printing Office, p. 127

US Tariff Commission (1970) Imports of Benzenoid Chemicals and Products, 1969, TC Publication 328, Washington DC, US Government Printing Office, p. 91

US Tariff Commission (1973) Imports of Benzenoid Chemicals and Products, 1972, TC Publication 601, Washington DC, US Government Printing Office, p. 95

Uyeta, M., Taue, S., Chikazawa, K. & Nishimoto, T. (1971) Pesticides translocated in food - organochlorine pesticides in the total diet. Shokuhin Eiseigaku Zasshi (J. Fd Hyg. Soc. Jap.), 12, 445

Uzoukwu, M. & Sleight, S.D. (1972) Effect of dieldrin in pregnant sows. J. amer. vet. Med. Ass., 1160, 1641

Vermeer, K. & Reynolds, L.M. (1971) Organochlorine residues in aquatic birds in the Canadian prairie provinces. Can. Fld-Nat., 84, 117

Versteeg, J.P.J. & Jager, K.W. (1973) Long-term occupational exposure to the insecticides aldrin, dieldrin, endrin and telodrin. Brit. J. industr. Med., 30, 201

Walker, A.I.T., Stevenson, D.E., Robinson, J., Thorpe, E. & Roberts, M. (1969) The toxicology and pharmacodynamics of dieldrin (HEOD): two-year oral exposure of rats and dogs. Toxicol. appl. Pharmacol., 15, 345

Walker, A.I.T., Thorpe, E., Robinson, J. & Baldwin, M.K. (1971) Toxicity studies on the photoisomerisation product of dieldrin. Meded. Fac. Landbauwetensch., 36, 398

Walker, A.I.T., Thorpe, E. & Stevenson, D.E. (1973) The toxicology of dieldrin (HEOD). I. Long-term oral toxicity studies in mice. Fd Cosmet. Toxicol., 11, 415

Walker, C.H., Hamilton, G.A. & Harrison, R.B. (1967) Organochlorine insecticide residues in wild birds in Britain. J. Sci. Fd Agric., 18, 123

Weil, L., Quentin, K.E. & Gitzowa, S. (1972) Zur Analytik der Pestizide im Wasser. IV. Kinetik der Pestizidanreicherung in Polyaethylen. Gas-Wasserfach Wasser-Abwasser, 113, 64

Wheatley, G.A. & Hardman, J.A. (1965) Indications of the presence of organochlorine insecticides in rainwater in central England. Nature (Lond.), 207, 486

Whetstone, R.R. (1964) Chlorocarbons and chlorohydrocarbons: chlorinated derivatives of cyclopentadiene. In: Kirk, R.E. & Othmer, D.F., eds., Encyclopedia of Chemical Technology, 2nd ed., New York, John Wiley & Sons, Vol. 5, p. 240

Wiemeyer, S.N., Mulhern, B.M., Ligas, F.J., Hensel, R.L., Mathisen, J.E., Robards, F.C. & Postupalsky, S. (1972) Residues of organochlorine pesticides, polychlorinated biphenyls and mercury in bald eagle eggs and changes in shell thickness, 1969 and 1970. Pest. Monit. J., 6, 50

Wiersma, G.B., Mitchell, W.G. & Stanford, C.L. (1972a) Pesticide residues in onions and soil - 1969. Pest. Monit. J., 5, 345

Wiersma, G.B., Taÿ, H. & Sand, P.F. (1972b) Pesticide residue levels in soils, FY 1969 - National Soils Monitoring Program. Pest. Monit. J., 6, 194

Wiersma, G.B., Taÿ, H. & Sand, P.F. (1972c) Pesticide residues in soil from eight cities - 1969. Pest. Monit. J., 6, 126

Williams, S. & Mills, P.A. (1964) Residues in milk of cows fed rations containing low concentrations of five chlorinated hydrocarbon pesticides. J. Ass. off. analyt. Chem., 47, 1124

Winnett, G. & Reed, J.P. (1968) Aldrin, dieldrin, endrin and chlordane persistence - a 3-year study. Pest. Monit. J., 2, 133

Wolfe, H.R., Durham, W.F. & Armstrong, J.F. (1963) Health hazards of the pesticides endrin and dieldrin: hazards in some agricultural uses in the Pacific Northwest. Arch. environm. Hlth, 6, 458

Wolfe, H.R., Durham, W.F. & Armstrong, J.F. (1967) Exposure of workers to pesticides. Arch. environm. Hlth, 14, 622

Zavon, M.R., Tye, R. & Stemmer, K. (1967) Effect of dieldrin insecticide on rhesus monkeys after three years of ingestion. Toxicol. appl. Pharmacol., 10, 391

ENDRIN

Endrin is the common name approved by the International Standards Organization (except in India and South Africa, where the name Mendrin is used) for 1,2,3,4,10,10-hexachloro-6,7-epoxy-1,4,4a,5,6,7,8,8a-octahydro-exo-1,4-exo-5,8-dimethanonaphthalene. Two reviews on this compound are available (FAO/WHO, 1965, 1971).

1. Chemical and Physical Data

1.1 Synonyms and trade names

Chem. Abstr. No.: 72-20-8

Compound 269; Experimental Insecticide 269; hexachloroepoxyoctahydro-endo,endo-dimethanonaphthalene; 1,2,3,4,10,10-hexachloro-6,7-epoxy-1,4,4a,5,6,7,8,8a-octahydro-endo,endo-1,4:5,8-dimethanonaphthalene; 1,2,3,4,10,10-hexachloro-6,7-epoxy-1,4,4a,5,6,7,8,8a-octahydro-endo-1,4-endo-5,8-dimethanonaphthalene; 1,2,3,4,10,10-hexachloro-6,7-epoxy-1,4,4a,5,6,7,8,8a-octahydro-1,4 endo,endo-5,8-dimethanonaphthalene; 1,2,3,4,10,10-hexachloro-6,7-epoxy-1,4,4a,5,6,7,8,8a-octahydro-1,4,5,8-endo-endo-dimethanonaphthalene; Mendrin

1.2 Chemical formula and molecular weight

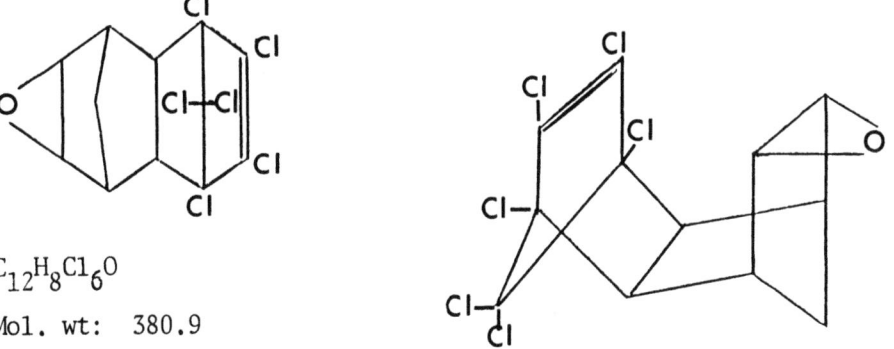

$C_{12}H_8Cl_6O$

Mol. wt: 380.9

1.3 Chemical and physical properties of the pure substance

(a) Description: White, crystalline solid

(b) Melting-point: Decomposes above 200°C

(c) <u>Solubility</u>: Soluble in acetone, benzene, carbon tetrachloride, hexane and xylene; practically insoluble in water

(d) <u>Volatility</u>: Vapour pressure is 2×10^{-7} mm Hg at $25°C$

(e) <u>Chemical reactivity</u>: Endrin is stable in the presence of most alkalis but rearranges to delta-keto endrin, shown below, in the presence of strong acids, in sunlight and when heated (Whetstone, 1964).

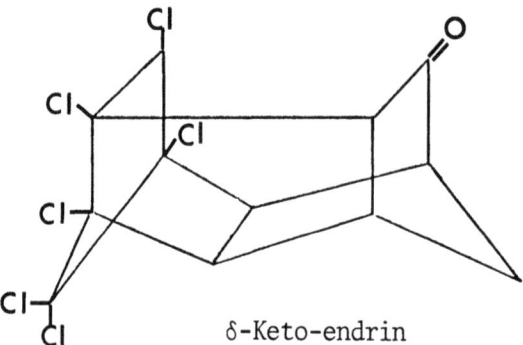

δ-Keto-endrin

1.4 Technical products and impurities

Technical endrin consists of cream to light-tan coloured, liquid-like crystals or powder with a mild chemical odour; it usually has a minimum purity of 95%. Endrin is available in the United States as a technical grade product containing 95% minimum active ingredient (equivalent to 95% hexachloro-epoxy-octahydro-<u>endo</u>,<u>endo</u>-dimethanonaphthalene) with 55-57% chlorine content, less than 0.4% free acid (as HCl) and less than 0.1% water (Frear, 1972; Whetstone, 1964). It is formulated into emulsifiable concentrates, dusts, granules and baits.

2. Production, Use, Occurrence and Analysis

Two review articles on endrin have appeared (Whetstone, 1964; Galley, 1970).

2.1 Production and use[1]

Endrin was first synthesized in around 1950 (Whetstone, 1964), and

---

[1] Data from Chemical Information Services, Stanford Research Institute, USA

commercial production in the US was first reported in 1953 (US Tariff Commission, 1954). Endrin, an isomer of dieldrin, is made by the epoxidation with peracetic acid of isodrin (prepared by the Diels-Alder addition of cyclopentadiene to hexachlorobicycloheptadiene) (Whetstone, 1964).

Only one or two companies in the US have manufactured endrin in any one year. Whetstone (1964) has estimated that 2.3-4.5 million kg of endrin were sold in the US in 1962, and another source has estimated that less than 450 thousand kg were produced in 1971 (Johnson, 1972).

Imports of endrin through the principal US customs districts were reported to have been nearly 21 thousand kg in 1972 (US Tariff Commission, 1973).

The following European countries were reported to be producing endrin in 1972 or 1973 (number of producing companies is given in parentheses): Belgium (1); France (1); Italy (1); and The Netherlands (1) (Chemical Information Services, Ltd., 1973; Ragno, 1972).

In 1972, Japan was reported to have 12 suppliers of endrin and endrin formulations, some of which may also have produced endrin (Chemical Daily Co., 1973), and imports were reported to have amounted to 72 thousand kg in 1970 (Hayashi, 1971).

The only known uses of endrin are as an insecticide, as an avicide and as a rodenticide (the first is believed to be the most important use). As of June 11, 1971 endrin was approved in the US for use on 7 agricultural crops (including 4 grains) and for use in the treatment of cotton seeds (with restrictions on the use of treated seeds) (US Environmental Protection Agency, 1971). As of August 1972 endrin was approved for use in the protection of forest seed against birds, mice and chipmunks, and for the control of birds on buildings and of mice in orchards (US Environmental Protection Agency, 1972).

Endrin usage in California, a major agricultural state, was reported to have been 4.2 thousand kg in 1971 (California Department of Agriculture, 1972) but only 600 kg in 1972 (California Department of Agriculture, 1973).

A general indication of possible uses of endrin or endrin + delta keto endrin combinations can be derived from the FAO/WHO recommended tolerances and practical residue limits for the following products: cottonseed, cottonseed oil, sweet corn, apples, wheat, barley, rice (husked and/or polished), sorghum, milk fat, poultry fat and eggs (FAO/WHO, 1973).

On July 3, 1973 the US Environmental Protection Agency proposed a list of toxic pollutants, which includes endrin (US Environmental Protection Agency, 1973). If this list is adopted, effluent standards restricting or prohibiting discharges of endrin into streams may come into effect.

The use of endrin has been banned in Switzerland (Anon., 1972) and in Italy. Its use will be permitted in the Federal Republic of Germany for the control of field-mice in fruit plantations until the end of 1974 (BBLF, 1972), and it has limited uses in the UK (UK Ministry of Agriculture, Fisheries and Food, 1973).

2.2 Occurrence

(a) Occupational exposure

During cropland spraying, concentrations in air ranged from trace amounts to 7.0 mg/m^3 (Kale & Dangwal, 1971). Potential dermal exposure during orchard spraying was calculated to have ranged from 2.5-3 mg/hr, and for respiratory exposure the amount was found to reach 0.01 mg/hr (Wolfe et al., 1963, 1967). During dusting of potatoes, levels of 18.5 mg/hr for dermal exposure and 0.41 mg/hr for respiratory exposure were found (Wolfe et al., 1963). During the spraying of row-crops, a dermal exposure of 0.15 mg/hr was found, but the respiratory exposure was below the limits of detection of the analytical method (Jegier, 1964).

(b) Air

Endrin could be detected in only 1 out of 9 localities of various sections of the US, the maximum level being 58.5 ng/m^3 (Stanley et al., 1971).

(c) Soil and water

Endrin residues are seldom found in soil. Concentrations in agricultural soils have been found to range from <0.01-0.5 ppm (Gish, 1970; Saha & Sumner, 1971; Wiersma et al., 1972a), and in 3 out of 8 cities average soil concentrations of <0.01 ppm have been detected (Wiersma et al., 1972b).

Endrin has rarely been found in surface water (Breidenbach et al., 1967; Brown & Nishioka, 1967; Lichtenberg et al., 1970; Manigold & Schulze, 1969); maximum values found were 0.1 µg/l (Lichtenberg et al., 1970) and <5 µg/l (Rowe et al., 1971).

(d) Animals

In oysters, a median value of <0.01 ppm has been detected (Bugg et al., 1967; Modin, 1969; Rowe et al., 1971).

(e) Food

Endrin is not stored in large amounts in plants and animal tissues and as a consequence has only rarely been found in food items. The residues in cottonseed, rice, sugar cane, grain and apples resulting from supervised trials are summarized in FAO/WHO (1971). In general, only very small amounts (<0.01-0.05 ppm) were found.

Cummings et al. (1967) fed diets containing between 0.05 and 0.45 ppm endrin to hens for 14 weeks and found residues ranging from 0.003-0.03 ppm in breast meat, and from 0.25-3.5 ppm in fat. Similar diets gave endrin residues of 0.03-0.32 ppm in eggs (Cummings et al., 1966). Saha (1969) summarizes the residues found in the milk of cows fed known amounts of endrin in their daily ration; the average amount (ppm) excreted in the milk/ppm intake ranged from 0.05-0.08.

In a series of analyses of total diets endrin was detected mainly in dairy products at levels of 0.002-0.003 ppm (Cummings, 1966). In meat, fish and poultry this substance was found from trace amounts to 0.001 ppm (Corneliussen, 1970; Cummings, 1966; Duggan et al., 1966). In vegetables, endrin has been found mostly in potatoes, maximum values ranging from 0.003-0.01 ppm (Corneliussen, 1969, 1970, 1972; Cummings, 1966; Duggan et al., 1967; Martin & Duggan, 1968). It was also found to be present in trace amounts in root, leafy and legume vegetables and fruits;

Bhalla et al. (1970) detected 0.06-0.38 ppm in fruits in India. Endrin has also been found in grains and cereals (0.003-0.004 ppm) and in oils (trace amounts-0.001 ppm) (Cummings, 1966; Duggan et al., 1967); in crude cottonseed oil produced by mills in Venezuela, Brazil, India and the US endrin residues ranged from <0.01-0.06 ppm (FAO/WHO, 1971). In cottonseed cakes, which are used as cattle feed concentrates, endrin concentrations ranged from <0.01-0.08 ppm (FAO/WHO, 1971).

In the US, Duggan & Lipscomb (1969) and Duggan & Corneliussen (1972) found that the total average intake from food ranged from about 0.01 µg/kg bw/day in 1965 to 0.0005 µg/kg bw/day in 1970. The 6-year average intake was 0.005 µg/kg bw/day.

An acceptable daily intake of 0-0.0002 mg/kg bw has been established by the Joint FAO/WHO Meeting on Pesticide Residues in Food (FAO/WHO, 1971).

In the US, a threshold limit value of 0.1 mg/m^3 for an 8-hour time-weighted average occupational exposure has been established (US Code of Federal Regulations, 1972).

2.3 Analysis

A general approach to the analysis of organochlorine pesticides has been given in the preamble (p. 16).

A gas chromatographic method for use on animal feed is described by Begliomini & Fravolini (1971), and a thin-layer chromatographic method by Mukherjee et al. (1971). In addition, a gel-permeation chromatographic method which requires little or no additional clean-up has been used on fish extracts (Stalling et al., 1972). A simple and rapid method for the determination of endrin residues in soil and water, sensitive at the 0.01 ppm level, has been described by Woodham et al. (1972). Chau et al. have published several papers dealing with the determination of endrin residues by the formation of derivatives: chromous chloride reduction followed by GLC analysis enables residues as low as 0.04 ppm to be determined (Chau & Cochrane, 1971). Photoproducts can be determined by silylation or acetylation, and levels of 0.02-0.03 ppm of these residues in 25 g fish sample extract or 0.01 ppb in 1 litre of water extract can be identified (Chau,

1972a). The use of derivative formation in a solid matrix enables as little as 1 ng of endrin to be confirmed in a cleaned-up sample extract (Chau, 1972b). In addition, Chau & Wilkinson (1972) have compared the separation characteristics of OV-101/OV-210 columns for organochlorine pesticides with particular reference to the separation of endrin and photoendrin.

Further references giving specific methods used for the analysis of endrin in various media can be found in the section on "Occurrence".

3. Biological Data Relevant to the Evaluation of Carcinogenic Risk to Man

3.1 Carcinogenicity and related studies in animals

(a) Oral administration

Mouse: (The Working Group was aware of an unpublished study in mice, some details of which were reported by FAO/WHO (1971).)

Rat: Six groups of 20 male and 20 female Carworth rats were administered diets containing endrin at concentrations of 0, 1, 5, 25, 50 or 100 ppm for 2 years. Survivors at 80 weeks included 12/80 rats given 50 or 100 ppm, 23/40 rats given 25 ppm, 28/40 given 5 ppm, 31/40 given 1 ppm and 28/40 in the control group. The incidence of neoplasia is stated to have been no greater among experimental animals than among controls, but no details are given (Treon et al., 1955).

Groups of 50 male and 50 female Osborne-Mendel rats were administered diets containing 2, 6 or 12 ppm endrin (technical 98%) for lifespan. In a control group containing 100 rats of each sex the mean survival time was 19.7 months in males and 19.5 months in females. In treated rats it ranged between 17.6 months in males given 12 ppm and 20.8 months in females given 2 ppm endrin. The proportion of tumour-bearing rats and the incidence of mammary tumours, lymphomas and other tumours in treated rats were similar to those observed in control animals. However, details of the time of appearance of tumours are not given. No liver-cell tumours were reported (Deichmann et al., 1970).

3.2 Other relevant biological data

(a) Metabolism and storage in animals

When ^{14}C-labelled endrin was fed to male and female rats, the males excreted 60% of the administered material in the faeces within the first 24 hours and the females only 39%. Less than 1% was excreted in the urine. Of the total radioactivity excreted in the faeces 70-75% occurred in the form of hydrophilic metabolites, the remainder was in unchanged endrin; 24 hours after the last dose only hydrophilic metabolites were excreted (Jager, 1970). When ^{14}C-labelled endrin was given orally and intravenously to rats, a major, more hydrophilic metabolite, the keto-analog of endrin, was identified in urine, and other hydrophilic metabolites were observed in trace amounts (Klein et al., 1968). Conversion of endrin to its metabolites occurs in the liver (Jager, 1970). When male rats with bile fistulas were given i.v. doses of ^{14}C-endrin (0.25 mg/kg bw), about 50% was excreted in the bile within 1 hour (Cole et al., 1970).

Oral administration of ^{14}C-endrin to rats in daily doses of 8 μg in peanut oil for 12 days resulted in equilibrium after 6 days. After 12 days, the spleen had the highest concentration, 3 ppm, the blood, 1.1 ppm, the skin and subcutaneous adipose tissue, 0.74 ppm, the peritoneal adipose tissue, 0.38 ppm and the brain, 0.25 ppm. Four days after cessation of feeding, male rats were found to have retained only 5.3% of the total radioactive material given and the females 15% (Klein et al., 1968).

Richardson et al. (1967) fed endrin to 9-month old dogs for 128 days at a level of 0.1 mg/kg bw/day. Blood samples were analyzed at weekly intervals, and concentrations from 0.002-0.008 ppm were found. At the end of the experiment concentrations in adipose tissue ranged from 0.3-0.8 ppm; heart, pancreas and muscle were at the lower end of this range, and the concentration in liver was 0.077-0.084 ppm; kidneys and lungs had similar concentrations. Very little endrin, as compared to other organochlorine insecticides, is stored in animals.

(b) Metabolism and storage in man

Low blood levels were found in 3 humans who recovered after accidental ingestion of endrin. In one case, the concentration of endrin in the blood 30 minutes after convulsions occurred was 0.053 ppm, and 20 hours later it was 0.038 ppm. The same patient excreted 0.02 ppm endrin in his urine during the next 24 hours (Coble et al., 1967). No residues were detected in plasma, adipose tissue and urine of workers occupationally exposed to endrin (Hayes & Curley, 1968).

3.3 Observations in man

(a) Studies on workers exposed to endrin

A study was undertaken in 1968 on 233 workers employed in a factory which had been manufacturing aldrin and dieldrin since 1954-1955, endrin since 1957 and telodrin during 1958-1965. Lengths of exposure ranged from 4-13.2 years (average, 7.6 years). One hundred and eighty-one workers were still employed by the same firm at the time of the study, and their average age was 41 years (range, 22-64). Only 2 deaths had occurred, and one had been caused by stomach cancer (Jager, 1970). The 52 workers who had left the company have been the subject of a subsequent report. Average age at the time of this survey was 47.4 years (range, 29-72), average occupational exposure was 6.6 years (4.0-12.3) and average time since end of exposure was 7.4 years (4.5-16). Only one death was recorded, and this had not been caused by cancer (Versteeg & Jager, 1973).

4. Comments on Data Reported and Evaluation

4.1 Animal data

In oral experiments in mice, insufficient details were available to allow an evaluation to be made.

Two feeding studies in rats were reported. One was negative, although the time when the tumours occurred in both treated and control groups was not given; the other provided no details of pathological studies and therefore cannot be evaluated.

4.2 Human data

The epidemiological study carried out on occupationally exposed workers does not allow any conclusions to be made concerning the existence of an excess risk of developing cancer.

5. References

Anon. (1972) Le DDT interdit en Suisse depuis le 1er avril 1972. Phytoma, 239, 37 (An English abstract is given in Health Aspects of Pesticides Abstract Bulletin, 72-2520)

BBLF (Biologische Bundesanstalt für Land- und Forstwirtschaft) (1972) Pflanzenschutzmittel-Verzeichnis, Merkblatt Nr. 1, 23. Auflage, April, Braunschweig, Federal Republic of Germany

Begliomini, A. & Fravolini, A. (1971) Residui di insetticidi nei mangimi. II. Identificazione e dosaggio gas cromatografico di insetticidi clorurati ed esteri fosforici in mangimi composti. Arch. vet. ital., 22, 109

Bhalla, J.S., Krueger, H.R., Bindra, O.S. & Deshmukh, S.N. (1970) Estimation of endrin residues in/on bhindi fruits by gas chromatography. Ind. J. Entomol., 32, 189

Breidenbach, A.W., Gunnerson, C.G., Kawahara, F.K., Lichtenberg, J.J. & Green, R.S. (1967) Chlorinated hydrocarbon pesticides in major river basins, 1957-65. Publ. Hlth Rep., 82, 139

Brown, E. & Nishioka, Y.A. (1967) Pesticides in selected western streams - a contribution to the national program. Pest. Monit. J., 1, ii, 38

Bugg, J.C., Jr, Higgins, J.E. & Robertson, E.A., Jr (1967) Chlorinated pesticide levels in the eastern oyster (Crassostrea virginica) from selected areas of the South Atlantic and Gulf of Mexico. Pest. Monit. J., 1, iii, 9

California Department of Agriculture (1972) Pesticide Use Report, 1971, Sacramento, p. 78

California Department of Agriculture (1973) Pesticide Use Report, 1972, Sacramento, pp. 85-86

Chau, A.S.Y. (1972a) Confirmation of pesticide residue identity. I. Derivative formation for the confirmation of photoproducts of endrin: hexachloro- and pentachloro-ketone pesticide residues by gas chromatography. J. Ass. off. analyt. Chem., 55, 519

Chau, A.S.Y. (1972b) Confirmation of pesticide residue identity. III. Derivative formation in solid matrix for the confirmation of endrin by gas chromatography. Bull. environm. Contam. Toxicol., 8, 169

Chau, A.S.Y. & Cochrane, W.P. (1971) Chromous chloride reductions. VI. Derivative formation for the simultaneous identification of heptachlor and endrin pesticide residues by gas chromatography. J. Ass. off. analyt. Chem., 54, 1124

Chau, A.S.Y. & Wilkinson, R.J. (1972) Some separation characteristics of an OV-101/OV-210 column for organochlorinated pesticides with particular reference to the separation of photoendrin and endrin. Bull. environm. Contam. Toxicol., 7, 93

Chemical Information Services, Ltd. (1973) Directory of West European Chemical Producers, Oceanside, NY

Coble, Y., Hildebrandt, P., Davis, J., Raasch, F. & Curley, A. (1967) Acute endrin poisoning. J. amer. med. Ass., 202, 489

Cole, J.F., Klevay, L.M. & Zavon, M.R. (1970) Endrin and dieldrin: a comparison of hepatic excretion in the rat. Toxicol. appl. Pharmacol., 16, 547

Corneliussen, P.E. (1969) Pesticide residues in total diet samples (IV). Pest. Monit. J., 2, 140

Corneliussen, P.E. (1970) Pesticide residues in total diet samples (V). Pest. Monit. J., 4, 89

Corneliussen, P.E. (1972) Pesticide residues in total diet samples (VI). Pest. Monit. J., 5, 313

Cummings, J.G. (1966) Pesticides in the total diet. Res. Rev., 16, 30

Cummings, J.G., Zee, K.T., Turner, V., Quinn, F. & Cook, R.E. (1966) Residues in eggs from low level feeding of five chlorinated hydrocarbon insecticides to hens. J. Ass. off. analyt. Chem., 49, 354

Cummings, J.G., Eidelman, M., Turner, V., Reed, D., Zee, K.T. & Cook, R.E. (1967) Residues in poultry tissues from low level feeding of five chlorinated hydrocarbon insecticides to hens. J. Ass. off. analyt. Chem., 50, 418

Deichmann, W.B., MacDonald, W.E., Blum, E., Bevilacqua, M., Radomski, J.L., Keplinger, M. & Balkus, M. (1970) Tumorigenicity of aldrin, dieldrin and endrin in the albino rat. Industr. Med. Surg., 39, 426

Duggan, R.E. & Corneliussen, P.E. (1972) Dietary intake of pesticide chemicals in the United States (III), June 1968-April 1970. Pest. Monit. J., 5, 331

Duggan, R.E. & Lipscomb, G.Q. (1969) Dietary intake of pesticide chemicals in the United States (II), June 1966-April 1968. Pest. Monit. J., 2, 153

Duggan, R.E., Barry, H.C. & Johnson, L.Y. (1966) Pesticide residues in total diet samples. Science, 151, 101

Duggan, R.E., Barry, H.C. & Johnson, L.Y. (1967) Pesticide residues in total diet samples (II). Pest. Monit. J., 1, ii, 2

FAO/WHO (1965) Evaluation of the toxicity of pesticide residues in food. FAO/PL: 1965/10/1; WHO/Food Add./27.65

FAO/WHO (1971) 1970 Evaluations of some pesticide residues in food. FAO/AGP/1970/M/12/1; WHO/Food Add./71.42, pp. 305-309, 312

FAO/WHO (1973) Pesticide residues in food. Report of the 1972 Joint FAO/WHO Meeting. Wld Hlth Org. techn. Rep. Ser., No. 525, p. 33

Frear, D.E.H., ed. (1972) Pesticide Handbook - Entoma, 24th ed., State College, Pennsylvania, College Science Publishers, p. 127

Galley, R.A.E. (1970) Chlorkohlenwasserstoffe: 4. Cyclodien-Insektizide. In: Wegler, R., ed., Chemie der Pflanzenschutz- und Schädlingsbekämpfungsmittel, Berlin, Heidelberg, New York, Springer-Verlag, 1, p. 163

Gish, C.D. (1970) Organochlorine insecticide residues in soils and soil invertebrates from agricultural lands. Pest. Monit. J., 3, 241

Hayashi, M. (1971) Residues of agricultural drugs and health of children. Shohni Hoken Kenkyu (Children Hlth Study), 30, 1

Hayes, W.J., Jr & Curley, A. (1968) Storage and excretion of dieldrin and related compounds. Effect of occupational exposure. Arch. environm. Hlth, 16, 155

Jager, K.W. (1970) Aldrin, dieldrin, endrin and telodrin. An epidemiological and toxicological study of long-term occupational exposure. Amsterdam, London, New York, Elsevier

Japan Chemical Week, ed. (1973) Japan Chemical Directory, Tokyo, The Chemical Daily Co., Ltd.

Jegier, Z. (1964) Health hazards in insecticide spraying of crops. Arch. environm. Hlth, 8, 670

Johnson, O. (1972) Pesticides '72. Chemical Week, June 21, p. 60

Kale, S.C. & Dangwal, S.K. (1971) Hazards during the use of pesticides/insecticides in agricultural farms. In: Proceedings of the Seminar on Pollution and the Human Environment, Bombay, 1970, Bombay, Bhabha Atomic Research Centre, pp. 192-204

Klein, W., Korte, F., Weisgerber, I., Kaul, R., Müller, W. & Djirsarai, A. (1968) Über den Metabolismus von Endrin, Heptachlor und Telodrin. Qdal. Pldt. Mater. veg. (Den Haag), 15, 225

Lichtenberg, J.J., Eichelberger, J.W., Dressman, R.C. & Longbottom, J.E. (1970) Pesticides in surface waters of the United States - a 5-year summary, 1964-68. Pest. Monit. J., 4, 71

Manigold, D.B. & Schulze, J.A. (1969) Pesticides in selected western streams - a progress report. Pest. Monit. J., 3, 124

Martin, R.J. & Duggan, R.E. (1968) Pesticide residues in total diet samples (III). Pest. Monit. J., 1, iv, 11

Modin, J.C. (1969) Chlorinated hydrocarbon pesticides in California bays and estuaries. Pest. Monit. J., 3, 1

Mukherjee, G., Mathew, T.V., Mukherjee, A.K. & Mitra, S.N. (1971) Identification and separation of chlorinated pesticides by TLC on magnesium hydroxide. J. Fd Sci. Technol., 8, 152

Ragno, M., ed. (1972) Repertorio Chimico Italiano, Industriale e Commerciale, Milano, Asiminum

Richardson, L.A., Lane, J.R., Gardner, W.S., Peeler, J.T. & Campbell, J.E. (1967) Relationship of dietary intake to concentration of dieldrin and endrin in dogs. Bull. environm. Contam. Toxicol., 2, 207

Rowe, D.R., Canter, L.W., Snyder, P.J. & Mason, J.W. (1971) Dieldrin and endrin concentrations in a Louisiana estuary. Pest. Monit. J., 4, 177

Saha, J.G. (1969) Significance of organochlorine insecticide residues in fresh plants as possible contaminants of milk and beef products. Res. Rev., 26, 89

Saha, J.G. & Sumner, A.K. (1971) Organochlorine insecticide residues in soil from vegetable farms in Saskatchewan. Pest. Monit. J., 5, 28

Stalling, D.L., Tindle, R.C. & Johnson, J.L. (1972) Clean-up of pesticide and polychlorinated biphenyl residues in fish extracts by gel permeation chromatography. J. Ass. off. analyt. Chem., 55, 32

Stanley, C.W., Barney, J.E., II, Helton, M.R. & Yobs, A.R. (1971) Measurement of atmospheric levels of pesticides. Environm. Sci. Technol., 5, 430

Treon, J.F., Cleveland, F.P. & Cappel, J. (1955) Toxicity of endrin for laboratory animals. J. agric. Fd Chem., 3, 842

UK Ministry of Agriculture, Fisheries and Food (1973) List of approved products and their uses for farmers and growers, London

US Code of Federal Regulations (1972) Washington DC, US Government Printing Office, 29 CFR. 1910.93

US Environmental Protection Agency (1971) EPA Compendium of Registered Pesticides, Washington DC, US Government Printing Office, pp. III-E-2.1 - III-E-2.3

US Environmental Protection Agency (1972) EPA Compendium of Registered Pesticides, Washington DC, US Government Printing Office, pp. IV-E-1.1 - IV-E-1.3

US Environmental Protection Agency (1973) Water pollution prevention and control. Proposed list of toxic pollutants, US Federal Register, Vol. 38, No. 129, Washington DC, US Government Printing Office, pp. 18044-18045

US Tariff Commission (1954) Synthetic Organic Chemicals, United States Production and Sales, 1953 Second Series, Report No. 194, Washington DC, US Government Printing Office, p. 134

US Tariff Commission (1973) Imports of Benzenoid Chemicals and Products, 1972, TC Publication 601, Washington DC, US Government Printing Office, p. 95

Versteeg, J.P.J. & Jager, K.W. (1973) Long-term occupational exposure to the insecticides aldrin, dieldrin, endrin and telodrin. Brit. J. industr. Med., 30, 201

Whetstone, R.R. (1964) Chlorocarbons and chlorohydrocarbons: chlorinated derivatives of cyclopentadiene. In: Kirk, R.E. & Othmer, D.F., eds, Encyclopedia of Chemical Technology, 2nd ed., New York, John Wiley & Sons, Vol. 5, pp. 240-252

Wiersma, G.B., Taï, H. & Sand, P.F. (1972a) Pesticide residue levels in soils, FY 1969 - National Soils Monitoring Program. Pest. Monit. J., 6, 194

Wiersma, G.B., Taï, H. & Sand, P.F. (1972b) Pesticide residues in soil from eight cities - 1969. Pest. Monit. J., 6, 126

Wolfe, H.R., Durham, W.F. & Armstrong, J.F. (1963) Health hazards of the pesticides endrin and dieldrin: hazards in some agricultural uses in the Pacific Northwest. Arch. environm. Hlth, 6, 458

Wolfe, H.R., Durham, W.F. & Armstrong, J.F. (1967) Exposure of workers to pesticides. Arch. environm. Hlth, 14, 622

Woodham, D.W., Loftis, C.D. & Collier, C.W. (1972) Identification of the gas chromatographic dieldrin and endrin peaks by chemical conversion. J. agric. Fd Chem., 20, 163

HEPTACHLOR

Heptachlor is the common name approved by the International Standards Organization for 1,4,5,6,7,8,8-heptachloro-3a,4,7,7a-tetrahydro-4,7-methano-indene. Several reviews on this compound are available (FAO/WHO, 1967, 1968, 1969, 1970, 1971).

1. Chemical and Physical Data

1.1 Synonyms and trade names

Chem. Abstr. No.: 76-44-8

Drinox; E-3314; ENT 15,152; H; 1,4,5,6,7,8,8a-heptachlorodicyclo-pentadiene; 3,4,5,6,7,8,8-heptachlorodicyclopentadiene; heptachloro-tetrahydro-endo-methanoindene; 1,4,5,6,7,8,8-heptachloro-3a,4,7,7a-tetrahydro-4,7-endo-methanoindene; 1,4,5,6,7,8,8-heptachloro-3a,4,7,7a-tetrahydro-4,7-methanoindene; heptachlorotetrahydro-4,7-methano-indene; 1(3a),4,5,6,7,8,8-heptachloro-3a(1),4,7,7a-tetrahydro-4,7-methanoindene; 3a,4,5,6,7,8,8-heptachloro-3a,4,7,7a-tetrahydro-4,7-methanoindene; 1,4,5,6,7,10,10-heptachloro-4,7,8,9-tetrahydro-4,7-methyleneindene; 1,4,5,6,7,10,10-heptachloro-4,7,8,9-tetrahydro-4,7-endo-methyleneindene; Heptamul; Velsicol 104

1.2 Chemical formula and molecular weight

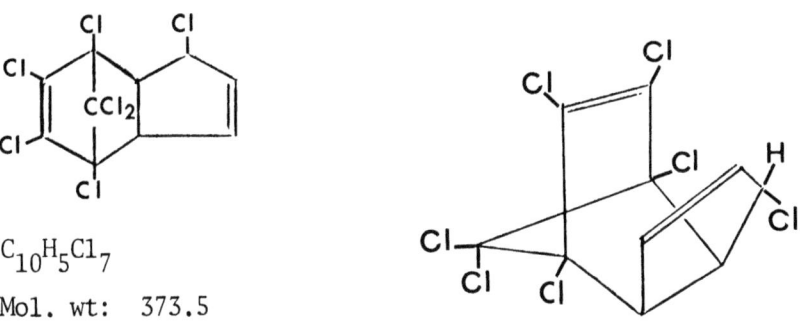

$C_{10}H_5Cl_7$

Mol. wt: 373.5

1.3 Chemical and physical properties of the pure substance

(a) Description: White, crystalline solid with a mild camphor odour

(b) Melting-point: 95-96°C

(c) Solubility: Soluble in (g/100 ml solvent at 27°C): acetone (75); benzene (106); carbon tetrachloride (112); cyclohexane (119); ethanol (4.5); xylene (102); and in water, 0.056 mg/l at 25-29°C

(d) Volatility: Vapour pressure is 3×10^{-4} mm Hg at 25°C

(e) Chemical reactivity: Heptachlor is readily converted to heptachlor epoxide

1.4 Technical products and impurities

The technical product (m.p., 46-74°C) is a light-tan, soft, waxy solid consisting of about 72% heptachlor and 28% related compounds (Martin, 1971). The technical product is also available in the form of emulsifiable concentrates, wettable powders and dusts (Berg, 1971).

Heptachlor epoxide

1.1 Synonyms and trade names

Chem. Abstr. No.: 1024-57-3

HE; 2,3,4,5,6,7,7-heptachloro-1a,1b,5,5a,6,6a-hexahydro-2,5-methano-2H-indeno[1,2-b]oxirene

1.2 Chemical formula and molecular weight

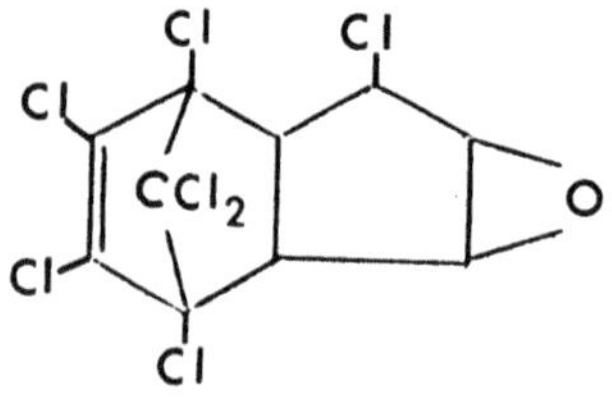

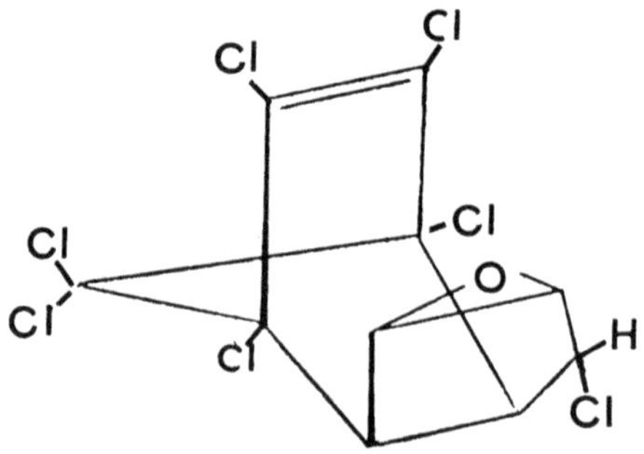

$C_{10}H_5Cl_7O$

Mol. wt: 389.35

1.3 Chemical and physical properties of the pure substance

Various spatial isomers of heptachlor epoxide are possible; two have been synthesized. The information given below relates to the compound formed in biological systems on the oxidation of heptachlor.

(a) <u>Description</u>: White, crystalline solid

(b) <u>Melting-point</u>: 159-160°C

(c) <u>Solubility</u>: In water, 0.2 mg/l at 25°C; soluble in fat and most organic solvents

(d) <u>Volatility</u>: Vapour pressure is 2.6×10^{-6} mm Hg at 20°C

(e) <u>Chemical reactivity</u>: Stable to concentrated sulphuric acid

2. Production, Use, Occurrence and Analysis

2.1 Production and use[1]

Heptachlor was first isolated from technical chlordane and first synthesized in about 1946 in both the United States and the Federal Republic of Germany (Lawless et al., 1972), however, commercial production in the US was not reported until 1953 (US Tariff Commission, 1954). Heptachlor is made by substitutive chlorination (sulphuryl chloride is the most efficient chlorinator) of chlordene in the presence of a catalyst (e.g., fullers' earth) which promotes substitution rather than addition of the chlorine (Whetstone, 1964). There is thought to be only one company manufacturing heptachlor in the US, and it has been estimated that this company probably sold less than 2.3 million kg of heptachlor in 1962 (Whetstone, 1964). Another source has estimated that 2.7 million kg of heptachlor were produced in 1971 (Johnson, 1972).

The only known use for heptachlor is as an insecticide. As of June 4, 1971 it was approved in the US for use on 22 agricultural crops (including several types of seed). Tolerances for combined residues of heptachlor and its oxidation product, heptachlor epoxide, were set at 0-0.1 ppm on many raw agricultural products, and restrictions were placed on the use of treated seeds (US Environmental Protection Agency, 1971).

---

[1] Data from Chemical Information Services, Stanford Research Institute, USA

The approved uses for heptachlor have been reviewed by the controlling US government agencies several times in the last few years, and these reviews have frequently resulted in restrictions on its application because of its persistence in the environment.

Heptachlor usage in California, a major agricultural state, was reported to have been only 424 kg in 1971 (California Department of Agriculture, 1972) and 1,239 kg in 1972 (over 98% of this was used for control of insects in structures) (California Department of Agriculture, 1973).

The widest application of heptachlor occurred in 1960, when it was used on forage, cereal and seed, vegetable, sugar beet and some nut crops. Subsequently, its use on vegetables, cereal seeds and soils was restricted in Canada, the US and Western Europe; when it has been applied to forage, grazing for that season is restricted (FAO/WHO, 1967).

Imports of heptachlor in Japan amounted to 133 thousand kg in 1970 (Hayashi, 1971).

Five per cent of the world's production of heptachlor in 1970 was used in Canada and the US. The percentage distribution of the remainder was as follows: Europe - 60%; Asia - 15%; South America - 15%; and Africa - 5% (FAO/WHO, 1971).

An indication of possible uses of heptachlor can be derived from the FAO/WHO recommended tolerances and practical limits on heptachlor in: pineapples (edible portion), milk and milk products, fat of meat and poultry, raw cereals, cotton seed, soybean oil (crude and edible), vegetables (including carrots, soybeans, tomatoes and sugar beets), citrus fruits and eggs (FAO/WHO, 1973).

Use of heptachlor in the Federal Republic of Germany for treatment of turnip seed will be allowed until the end of 1974 (BBLF, 1972); and its use has been banned in Switzerland (EFOWG; EFLP; SFRA, 1972, 1973/74), in the USSR (Melnikov & Shevchenko, 1971) and in Italy.

2.2 Occurrence

(a) Air

During an extensive programme in which the ambient air in various parts of the US was monitored, heptachlor could be detected in only 2 out of 9 localities at maximum levels of 19.2 and 2.3 ng/m^3, while no heptachlor epoxide was found in any of the samples (Stanley et al., 1971). In dust samples, Cohen & Pinkerton (1966) found concentrations of 0.04 ppm heptachlor epoxide.

(b) Soil and water

Many studies have been made of the heptachlor and heptachlor epoxide residue levels in agricultural soils (Gish, 1970; Saha & Sumner, 1971; Sand et al., 1972; Seal et al., 1967; Trautmann et al., 1968; Wiersma et al., 1972a,b), and average residue levels found ranged from 0.01-0.2 ppm heptachlor and/or heptachlor epoxide. The average soil concentration in 8 cities ranged from <0.01-0.02 ppm heptachlor and from <0.01-0.05 ppm heptachlor epoxide (Wiersma et al., 1972c).

Supervised applications of these two substances gave the following results: applications of 1-1.6 lb/acre heptachlor left no residues 15 months later; 2 lb/acre left 0.26-0.47 ppm heptachlor + heptachlor epoxide one year later; 3 lb/acre left 0.21-0.40 ppm 4 months later and 0.18-0.32 ppm one year later; and 6 lb/acre left 0.49-3.61 ppm 4 months later and 0.63-2.24 ppm one year later (FAO/WHO, 1971). Loam soil treated for 5 years with 5 lb/acre/year contained 4.6% of the applied heptachlor 5 years after cessation of treatment; thus the mean residue level in soil was 0.70 ppm heptachlor + heptachlor epoxide and in carrots 0.413 ppm (Lichtenstein et al., 1970). All other fruits or vegetables grown on treated soils showed none or negligible quantities of these compounds (FAO/WHO, 1971).

Heptachlor has rarely been found in surface waters, and then only in small quantities: 5-30 ppt for heptachlor and/or 5-40 ppt for heptachlor epoxide (Brown & Nishioka, 1967; Hannon et al., 1970; Herzel, 1972).

(c) Animals and plants

Heptachlor and/or its epoxide accumulate in body fat, the epoxide being more persistent than the parent compound. Heptachlor epoxide has been found in adipose tissue of fish and birds, in liver, brain and muscle of birds, and in insects, algae, plankton and birds eggs (FAO/WHO, 1967).

Fish can accumulate 0.008 mg/kg bw heptachlor + heptachlor epoxide from concentrations of 0.00006 mg/l in water (Hannon et al., 1970). Residues found in whole fish have ranged from <0.01-0.026 ppm heptachlor + heptachlor epoxide (Hannon et al., 1970; Henderson et al., 1969), and in fatty tissue from <0.01-0.8 ppm (Cole et al., 1967; Hannon et al., 1970). In oysters, median values of <0.01 ppm heptachlor and <0.01 ppm heptachlor epoxide have been found (Bugg et al., 1967).

Heptachlor epoxide has been detected in both domestic and wild bird species (Greichus et al., 1968; Linder & Dahlgren, 1970; Martin & Nickerson, 1972; Mulhern et al., 1970; Reichel et al., 1969); concentrations of heptachlor epoxide in fatty tissues were generally ten times higher than those in liver (0.3-3.0 ppm) or brain (0.3-0.6 ppm), and lower concentrations were found in breast muscle (0.1-1.4 ppm) (Walker et al., 1967).

In the carcasses of eagles, 0.06-0.08 ppm heptachlor epoxide have been detected (Mulhern et al., 1970; Reichel et al., 1969); and in pheasant fat, 0-0.66 ppm heptachlor epoxide have been found (Greichus et al., 1968; Linder & Dahlgren, 1970). Average concentrations of heptachlor epoxide in eagle eggs ranged from 0.02-0.08 ppm (Krantz et al., 1970; Wiemeyer et al., 1972), and concentrations in eggs of sea birds ranged from 0.01-0.9 ppm (Vermeer & Reynolds, 1971).

(d) Food

As the formation of heptachlor epoxide is relatively rapid, it is this compound which is most often detected. In the US and the UK, a series of analyses of total diets has been carried out (Abbott et al., 1969; Corneliussen, 1969, 1970, 1972; Cummings, 1966; Duggan & Corneliussen, 1972; Duggan & Lipscomb, 1969; Duggan & Weatherwax, 1967; Duggan et al., 1966, 1967, 1971; Martin & Duggan, 1968): heptachlor epoxide was found to be present in very small amounts in dairy products and meat, fish and poultry and in trace amounts in vegetables, fruits, oils and cereals.

In meat, fish and poultry maximum values of heptachlor epoxide found ranged from 0.06 ppm (Cummings, 1966) to 0.1 ppm (Corneliussen, 1972). Dairy products are contaminated mostly through feed, and the residues found are almost entirely heptachlor expoxide. Many data on controlled feeding of heptachlor and/or heptachlor epoxide have been reported, and these are summarized by Saha (1969) and in FAO/WHO (1971). In cows fed 5 or 20 ppb heptachlor epoxide daily for 27 days, up to 2.9 ppb and 4.4 ppb, respectively, were detected in the milk (Hardee et al., 1964); thus, since crops grown in heptachlor-treated soils or crops sprayed with heptachlor may have similar residues and be used as cattle feed, milk may be contaminated with similar small amounts of heptachlor epoxide (Saha, 1969).

In Canada, an average level of 0.001 ppm has been found in milk fat (Frank et al., 1970), and 0.0036 ppm heptachlor epoxide and 0.002 ppm heptachlor have been reported in the US (Duggan, 1967). In total diet studies in the US, maximum values for heptachlor epoxide ranged from 0.02 ppm (Cummings, 1966) to 0.05 ppm (Corneliussen, 1969, 1970, 1972).

In human milk, average concentrations ranging from traces to 0.008 ppm heptachlor epoxide have been detected (Curley & Kimbrough, 1969; Heyndrickx & Maes, 1969; Luquet et al., 1972; Ritcey et al., 1972). Kroger (1972) found an average of 0.16 ppm in human milk fat.

In the UK, the calculated amount of heptachlor epoxide in the total diet was generally less than 0.0005 mg/kg (ppm) (Abbott et al., 1969); heptachlor was not detected.

In the US, the average total daily intake of heptachlor from food has been reported to have ranged from 0.003 µg/kg bw/day in 1965 to 0.0001 µg/kg bw/day in 1970, with a 6-year average of 0.001 µg/kg bw/day. The total intake of heptachlor epoxide ranged from 0.03 µg/kg bw/day in 1965 to 0.02 µg/kg bw/day in 1970, with a 6-year average of 0.03 µg/kg bw/day (Duggan & Corneliussen, 1972).

An acceptable daily intake of 0-0.0005 mg/kg bw has been established for heptachlor (FAO/WHO, 1971).

In the US a threshold limit value of 0.5 mg/m^3 has been established for an 8-hour time-weighted average occupational exposure (US Code of Federal Regulations, 1972).

2.3 Analysis

A general approach to the analysis of organochlorine pesticides is given in the preamble (p. 16).

A rapid gas-liquid chromatographic method for confirming the presence of heptachlor epoxide has been reported by Conder et al. (1972), and a thin-layer chromatographic method for heptachlor is described by Mukherjee et al. (1971). A system employing support-bonded silicones on chromosorb has been developed for trapping organic vapours from air (Aue & Teli, 1971).

The presence of heptachlor residues can be confirmed by the formation of derivatives which are then determined by GLC (Chau & Cochrane, 1971; Chau & Lanouette, 1972; Cochrane & Chau, 1970). Heptachlor in waste water has been separated from sulphur and determined by the same method (Baird et al., 1973). A specific enzyme inhibition method for the determination of four chlorinated insecticides including heptachlor, in soils, has been developed by Nash et al. (1973).

Further analytical methods used for detection in various other media, such as air, water, food, etc., can be found in the references cited in the section on "Occurrence".

3. Biological Data Relevant to the Evaluation of Carcinogenic Risk to Man

3.1 Carcinogenicity and related studies in animals

(a) Oral administration

Mouse: An experiment was carried out in mice by the US Food and Drug Administration and its results were considered positive for tumour induction (US Department of Health, Education & Welfare, 1969). (These results have **not** been published or summarized in any publication available to the Working Group, thus it was not possible to express any opinion thereon.)

Rat: Five unpublished long-term experiments, in which heptachlor and/or heptachlor epoxide were fed in the diet to rats, have been summarized by the Joint FAO/WHO Expert Committee on pesticide residues. In three of these studies, in which groups of up to 40 rats received diets containing up to 12.5 ppm of the test material for at least 2 years, no increase in tumour incidence attributable to treatment was said to occur. Tumour incidence was not mentioned in a fourth test, although an increase in liver weight in animals receiving 10 and 20 ppm heptachlor was found.

In one study, heptachlor was fed at concentrations of 0.5, 2.5, 5, 7.5 and 10 ppm to CNFN rats. Survival rates were not reported. Although, when groups were considered together, there was an increase in the incidence of tumour-bearing animals (8/23 in male and 13/24 in female controls, as compared with 65/114 in male and 92/114 in female test animals), it did not appear likely that a significant dose-response relationship existed either for total or for hepatic tumours. Most tumours were located in endocrine organs; liver tumours were found in 7 male and 12 female test animals but in no control animals (FAO/WHO, 1967).

3.2 Other relevant biological data

(a) Metabolism and storage in animals

Rats and rabbits metabolize intravenously injected heptachlor to the epoxide (for structure see section 1.2) and to 4,5,6,7,8,8-hexachloro-1-exo-hydroxy-6,7-exo-epoxy-1,2,3a,4,7,7a-hexahydro-1,4-endo-methylene-indene (1)[*] (Klein et al., 1968). Another faecal metabolite (2)[*] was isolated from rats fed 10 ppm heptachlor epoxide for 30 days (Matsumura & Nelson, 1971).

Rats fed heptachlor stored heptachlor epoxide in their adipose tissue: at a dietary level of 30 ppm maximum concentrations were found in adipose tissue within 2-4 weeks. Twelve weeks after exposure to heptachlor was discontinued, heptachlor epoxide had completely disappeared from adipose tissue (Radomski & Davidow, 1953). Steers fed heptachlor and heptachlor

---

[*] For structure see page 182.

1-HYDROXY–CHLORDENE EPOXIDE (1)

FAECAL METABOLITE (2)

epoxide stored only heptachlor epoxide in their adipose tissue (Bovard et al., 1971); and similar results were obtained in dogs fed heptachlor alone (Davidow & Radomski, 1953).

(b) Metabolism and storage in man

Trace amounts of heptachlor epoxide have been found in the adipose tissue of the general population in most countries (Abbott et al., 1968, 1972; Curley et al., 1973; Davies et al., 1971; Edwards, 1970; Egan et al., 1965; Fournier et al., 1972; Hayes et al., 1965; Wassermann et al., 1970, 1972a,b,c). Maximum levels were reported in 1970 in France (0.28-0.36 ppm) (Fournier et al., 1972). In the US levels of 0.24 ppm were found in 1964 (Hayes et al., 1965), which had decreased to 0.05 ppm in 1969 (Davies et al., 1971).

Heptachlor epoxide is also found in the blood and fat of stillborn infants (levels of 0.2-0.3 ppm were found in fat), indicating transplacental transfer to the foetus (Curley et al., 1969; Wassermann et al., 1972a,c; Zavon et al., 1969). It is also excreted in human milk (Curley & Kimbrough, 1969). For additional data see table in appendix p. 224.

3.3 Observations in man

(a) Concentration of heptachlor in tissues of terminal patients

The average concentrations of heptachlor epoxide in fat, liver and brain did not differ significantly between cancerous and control patients (Radomski et al., 1968).

4. Comments on Data Reported and Evaluation

4.1 Animal data

Reports of tests on heptachlor and/or its epoxide were available only in rats by the oral route, and all studies have been inadequately reported. One of five experiments suggest hepatocarcinogenicity, but this was not reproduced in the other experiments within the same dose range. In view of incomplete reporting no conclusions could be reached.

4.1 _Human data_

No epidemiological studies were available to the Working Group. Patients with cancer did not show higher concentrations of heptachlor epoxide in fat tissues and liver than did control patients.

5. References

Abbott, D.C., Goulding, R. & Tatton, J.O'G. (1968) Organochlorine pesticide residues in human fat in Great Britain. Brit. med. J., iii, 146

Abbott, D.C., Holmes, D.C. & Tatton, J.O'G. (1969) Pesticide residues in the total diet in England and Wales, 1966-67. II. Organochlorine pesticide residues in the total diet. J. Sci. Fd Agric., 20, 245

Abbott, D.C., Collins, G.B. & Goulding, R. (1972) Organochlorine pesticide residues in human fat in the United Kingdom, 1969-71. Brit. med. J., ii, 553

Aue, W.A. & Teli, P.M. (1971) Sampling of air pollutants with support-bonded chromatographic phases. J. Chromat., 62, 15

Baird, R.B., Carmona, L.G. & Kuo, C.L. (1973) Gas-liquid chromatographic separation of sulfur from chlorinated pesticide residues in wastewater samples. Bull. environm. Contam. Toxicol., 9, 108

BBLF (Biologische Bundesanstalt für Land- und Forstwirtschaft) (1972) Pflanzenschutzmittel-Verzeichnis, Merkblatt Nr. 1, 23. Auflage, April, Braunschweig, Federal Republic of Germany

Berg, G.L., ed. (1971) Farm Chemicals Handbook, Willoughby, Ohio, Meister, p. D207

Bovard, K.P., Fontenot, J.P. & Priode, B.M. (1971) Accumulation and dissipation of heptachlor residues in fattening steers. J. Animal Sci., 33, 127

Brown, E. & Nishioka, Y.A. (1967) Pesticides in selected western streams - a contribution to the national program. Pest. Monit. J., 1, ii, 38

Bugg, J.C., Jr, Higgins, J.E. & Robertson, E.A., Jr (1967) Chlorinated pesticide levels in the eastern oyster (Crassostrea virginica) from selected areas of the South Atlantic and Gulf of Mexico. Pest. Monit. J., 1, iii, 9

California Department of Agriculture (1972) Pesticide Use Report, 1971, Sacramento, p. 90

California Department of Agriculture (1973) Pesticide Use Report, 1972, Sacramento, p. 99

Chau, A.S.Y. & Cochrane, W.P. (1971) Chromous chloride reductions. VI. Derivative formation for the simultaneous identification of heptachlor and endrin pesticide residues by gas chromatography. J. Ass. off. analyt. Chem., 54, 1124

Chau, A.S.Y. & Lanouette, M. (1972) Confirmation of pesticide residue identity. II. Derivative formation in solid matrix for the confirmation of DDT, DDD, methoxychlor, perthane, cis- and trans-chlordane, heptachlor and heptachlor epoxide pesticide residues by gas chromatography. J. Ass. off. analyt. Chem., 55, 1058

Cochrane, W.P. & Chau, A.S.Y. (1970) Use of chromous chloride for the confirmation of heptachlor residues by derivatization. Bull. environm. Contam. Toxicol., 5, 251

Cohen, J.M. & Pinkerton, C. (1966) Widespread translocation of pesticides by air transport and rainout. Organic Pesticides in the Environment, Adv. Chem. Ser., 60, 163

Cole, H., Bradford, A., Barry, D., Baumgarner, P. & Frear, D.E.H. (1967) Pesticides in hatchery trout - differences between species and residue levels occurring in commercial fish food. Pest. Monit. J., 1, ii, 35

Conder, D.W., Oloffs, P.C. & Szeto, Y.S. (1972) GLC separation of heptachlor epoxide, oxychlordane, α- and γ-chlordane. Bull. environm. Contam. Toxicol., 7, 33

Corneliussen, P.E. (1969) Pesticide residues in total diet samples (IV). Pest. Monit. J., 2, 140

Corneliussen, P.E. (1970) Pesticide residues in total diet samples (V). Pest. Monit. J., 4, 89

Corneliussen, P.E. (1972) Pesticide residues in total diet samples (VI). Pest. Monit. J., 5, 313

Cummings, J.G. (1966) Pesticides in the total diet. Res. Rev., 16, 30

Curley, A. & Kimbrough, R.D. (1969) Chlorinated hydrocarbon insecticides in plasma and milk of pregnant and lactating women. Arch. environm. Hlth, 18, 156

Curley, A., Copeland, M.F. & Kimbrough, R.D. (1969) Chlorinated hydrocarbon insecticides in organs of stillborn and blood of newborn babies. Arch. environm. Hlth, 19, 628

Curley, A., Burse, V.W., Jennings, R.W., Villanueva, E.C., Tomatis, L. & Akazaki, K. (1973) Chlorinated hydrocarbon pesticides and related compounds in adipose tissue from people of Japan. Nature (Lond.), 242, 338

Davidow, B. & Radomski, J.L. (1953) Isolation of an epoxide metabolite from fat tissues of dogs fed heptachlor. J. Pharmacol. exp. Ther., 107, 259

Davies, J.E., Edmundson, W.F., Maceo, A., Irvin, G.L., III, Cassady, J. & Barquet, A. (1971) Reduction of pesticide residues in human adipose tissue with diphenylhydantoin. Fd Cosmet. Toxicol., 9, 413

Duggan, R.E. (1967) Chlorinated pesticide residues in fluid milk and other dairy products in the United States. Pest. Monit. J., 1, iii, 2

Duggan, R.E. & Corneliussen, P.E. (1972) Dietary intake of pesticide chemicals in the United States (III), June 1968-April 1970. Pest. Monit. J., 5, 331

Duggan, R.E. & Lipscomb, G.Q. (1969) Dietary intake of pesticide chemicals in the United States (II), June 1966-April 1968. Pest. Monit. J., 2, 153

Duggan, R.E. & Weatherwax, J.R. (1967) Dietary intake of pesticide chemicals. Science, 157, 1006

Duggan, R.E., Barry, H.C. & Johnson, L.Y. (1966) Pesticide residues in total diet samples. Science, 151, 101

Duggan, R.E., Barry, H.C. & Johnson, L.Y. (1967) Pesticide residues in total diet samples (II). Pest. Monit. J., 1, ii, 2

Duggan, R.E., Lipscomb, G.Q., Cox, E.L., Heatwole, R.E. & Kling, R.C. (1971) Pesticide residue levels in foods in the United States from July 1, 1963 to June 30, 1969. Pest. Monit. J., 5, 73

Edwards, C.A., ed. (1970) Pesticide residues in human beings. In: Persistent pesticides in the environment, Cleveland, Ohio, CRC Press, p. 49

EFOWG; EFLP; SFRA (Eidg. Forschungsanstalt für Obst-, Wein- und Gartenbau, Wädenswil; Eidg. Forschungsanstalt für landwirtschaftlichen Pflanzenbau, Zürich-Reckenholz; Station fédérale de recherches agronomiques, Lausanne) (1972; 1973/4) Pflanzenschutzmittel-Verzeichnis, Bern, Eidg. Drucksachen- und Materialzentrale

Egan, H., Goulding, R., Roburn, J. & Tatton, J.O'G. (1965) Organochlorine pesticide residues in human fat and human milk. Brit. med. J., ii, 66

FAO/WHO (1967) Evaluations of some pesticide residues in food. FAO/PL: CP/15; WHO/Food Add./67.32

FAO/WHO (1968) 1967 Evaluations of some pesticide residues in food. FAO/PL/1967/M/11/1; WHO/Food Add./68.30

FAO/WHO (1969) 1968 Evaluations of some pesticide residues in food. FAO/PL/1968/M/9/1; WHO/Food Add./69.35

FAO/WHO (1970) 1969 Evaluations of some pesticide residues in food. FAO/PL/1969/M/17/1; WHO/Food Add./70.38

FAO/WHO (1971) 1970 Evaluations of some pesticide residues in food. FAO/AGP/1970/M/12/1; WHO/Food Add./71.42

FAO/WHO (1973) Pesticide residues in food. Report of the 1972 Joint FAO/WHO Meeting. Wld Hlth Org. techn. Rep. Ser., No. 525

Fournier, E., Treich, I., Campagne, L. & Capelle, N. (1972) Pesticides organochlorés dans le tissu adipeux d'êtres humains en France. Europ. J. Toxicol., 5, 11

Frank, R., Braun, H.E. & McWade, J.W. (1970) Chlorinated hydrocarbon residues in the milk supply of Ontario, Canada. Pest. Monit. J., 4, 31

Gish, C.D. (1970) Organochlorine insecticide residues in soils and soil invertebrates from agricultural lands. Pest. Monit. J., 3, 241

Greichus, Y.A., Greichus, A. & Reider, E.G. (1968) Insecticide residues in grouse and pheasant of South Dakota. Pest. Monit. J., 2, 90

Hannon, M.R., Greichus, Y.A., Applegate, R.L. & Fox, A.C. (1970) Ecological distribution of pesticides in Lake Poinsett, South Dakota. Trans. amer. Fish. Soc., 99, 496

Hardee, D.D., Gutenmann, W.H., Keenan, G.I., Gyrisco, G.G., Lisk, D.J., Fox, F.H., Trimberger, G.W. & Holland, R.F. (1964) Residues of heptachlor epoxide and telodrin in milk from cows fed at part per billion insecticide levels. J. econ. Entomol., 56, 404

Hayashi, M. (1971) Residues of agricultural drugs and health of children. Shohni Hoken Kenkyu (Children Hlth Study), 30, 1

Hayes, W.J., Jr, Dale, W.E. & Burse, V.W. (1965) Chlorinated hydrocarbon pesticides in the fat of people in New Orleans. Life Sci., 4, 1611

Henderson, C., Johnson, W.L. & Inglis, A. (1969) Organochlorine insecticide residues in fish (National Pesticide Monitoring Program). Pest. Monit. J., 3, 145

Herzel, F. (1972) Organochlorine insecticides in surface waters in Germany - 1970 and 1971. Pest. Monit. J., 6, 179

Heyndrickx, A. & Maes, R. (1969) The excretion of chlorinated hydrocarbon insecticides in human mother milk. J. Pharm. belg., 24, 459

Johnson, O. (1972) Pesticides '72. Chemical Week, July 26, p. 19

Klein, W., Korte, F., Weisgerber, I., Kaul, R., Mueller, W. & Djirsarai, A. (1968) Uber den Metabolismus von Endrin, Heptachlor und Telodrin. Qdal. Pldt. Mater. veg. (Den Haag), 15, 225

Krantz, W.C., Mulhern, B.M., Bagley, G.E., Sprunt, A., IV, Ligas, F.J. & Robertson, W.B., Jr (1970) Organochlorine and heavy metal residues in bald eagle eggs. Pest. Monit. J., 4, 136

Kroger, M. (1972) Insecticide residues in human milk. J. Pediat., 80, 401

Lawless, E.W., Rumker, R. & Furguson, T.L. (1972) The Pollution Potential in Pesticide Manufacturing. Pesticide Study Series 5, Technical Studies Report TS-00-72-04, Environmental Protection Agency, Washington DC, US Government Printing Office

Lichtenstein, E.P., Schulz, K.R., Fuhremann, T.W. & Liang, T.T. (1970) Degradation of aldrin and heptachlor in field soils during a ten-year period. Translocation into crops. J. agric. Fd Chem., 18, 100

Linder, R.L. & Dahlgren, R.B. (1970) Occurrence of organochlorine insecticides in pheasants of South Dakota. Pest. Monit. J., 3, 227

Luquet, F.M., Goursaud, J. & Gaudier, B. (1972) Etude de la pollution des laits humains par les résidus de pesticides. Path. Biol., 20, 137

Martin, H., ed. (1971) Pesticide Manual. Basic Information on the Chemicals used as Active Components of Pesticides, 2nd ed., Ombersley, British Crop Protection Council, p. 268

Martin, R.J. & Duggan, R.E. (1968) Pesticide residues in total diet samples (III). Pest. Monit. J., 1, iv, 11

Martin, W.E. & Nickerson, P.R. (1972) Organochlorine residues in starlings - 1970. Pest. Monit. J., 6, 33

Matsumura, F. & Nelson, J.O. (1971) Identification of the major metabolic product of heptachlor epoxide in rat feces. Bull. environm. Contam. Toxicol., 5, 489

Melnikov, N.H. & Shevchenko, M.G. (1971) Hygienic normalization of pesticide residues and their tolerance levels in foodstuffs in the USSR. Res. Rev., 35, 1

Mukherjee, G., Mathew, T.V., Mukherjee, A.K. & Mitra, S.N. (1971) Identification and separation of chlorinated pesticides by TLC on magnesium hydroxide. J. Fd Sci. Technol., 8, 152

Mulhern, B.M., Reichel, W.L., Locke, L.N., Lamont, T.G., Belisle, A., Cromartie, E., Bagley, G.E. & Prouty, R.M. (1970) Organochlorine residues and autopsy data from bald eagles, 1966-68. Pest. Monit. J., 4, 141

Nash, R.G., Harris, W.G., Ensor, P.D. & Woolson, E.A. (1973) Comparative extraction of chlorinated hydrocarbon insecticides from soils 20 years after treatment. J. Ass. off. analyt. Chem., 56, 728

Radomski, J.L. & Davidow, B. (1953) The metabolite of heptachlor: its estimation, storage and toxicity. J. Pharmacol. exp. Ther., 107, 266

Radomski, J.L., Deichmann, W.B. & Clizer, E.E. (1968) Pesticide concentrations in the liver, brain and adipose tissue of terminal hospital patients. Fd Cosmet. Toxicol., 10, 209

Reichel, W.L., Cromartie, E., Lamont, T.G., Mulhern, B.M. & Prouty, R.M. (1969) Pesticide residues in eagles. Pest. Monit. J., 3, 142

Ritcey, W.R., Savary, G. & McCully, K.A. (1972) Organochlorine insecticide residues in human milk, evaporated milk and some milk substitutes in Canada. Canad. J. publ. Hlth, 63, 125

Saha, J.G. (1969) Significance of organochlorine insecticide residues in fresh plants as possible contaminants of milk and beef products. Res. Rev., 26, 89

Saha, J.G. & Sumner, A.K. (1971) Organochlorine insecticide residues in soil from vegetable farms in Saskatchewan. Pest. Monit. J., 5, 28

Sand, P.F., Wiersma, G.B. & Landry, J.L. (1972) Pesticide residues in sweet potatoes and soil - 1969. Pest. Monit. J., 5, 342

Seal, W.L., Dawsey, L.H. & Cavin, G.E. (1967) Monitoring for chlorinated hydrocarbon pesticides in soil and root crops in the eastern states in 1965. Pest. Monit. J., 1, iii, 22

Stanley, C.W., Barney, J.E., II, Helton, M.R. & Yobs, A.R. (1971) Measurement of atmospheric levels of pesticides. Environm. Sci. Technol., 5, 430

Trautmann, W.L., Chesters, G. & Pionke, H.B. (1968) Organochlorine insecticide composition of randomly selected soils from nine states - 1967. Pest. Monit. J., 2, 93

US Code of Federal Regulations (1972) Washington DC, US Government Printing Office, 29 CFR 1910.83

US Department of Health, Education and Welfare (1969) Report of the Secretary's Commission on Pesticides and their Relationship to Environmental Health, Washington DC, US Government Printing Office

US Environmental Protection Agency (1971) EPA Compendium of Registered Pesticides, Washington DC, US Government Printing Office, pp. III-H-1.1 - III-H-1.4

US Tariff Commission (1954) Synthetic Organic Chemicals, United States Production and Sales, 1953 Second Series, Report No. 194, Washington DC, US Government Printing Office, p. 134

Vermeer, K. & Reynolds, L.M. (1971) Organochlorine residues in aquatic birds in the Canadian prairie provinces. Canad. Fld-Nat., 84, 117

Walker, C.H., Hamilton, G.A. & Harrison, R.B. (1967) Organochlorine insecticide residues in wild birds in Britain. J. Sci. Fd Agric., 18, 123

Wassermann, M., Wassermann, D. & Lazarovici, S. (1970) Present state of the storage of the organochlorine insecticides in the general population of South Africa. South Afr. med. J., 44, 646

Wassermann, M., Nogueira, D.P., Tomatis, L., Athie, E., Wassermann, D., Djavaherian, M. & Guttel, C. (1972a) Storage of organochlorine insecticides in people of Sao Paulo, Brazil. Industr. Med., 41, 22

Wassermann, M., Rogoff, M.G., Tomatis, L., Day, N.E., Wassermann, D., Djavaherian, M. & Guttel, C. (1972b) Storage of organochlorine insecticides in the adipose tissue of people in Kenya. Ann. Soc. belge Méd. trop., 52, 509

Wassermann, M., Sofoluwe, G.O., Tomatis, L., Day, N.E., Wassermann, D. & Lazarovici, S. (1972c) Storage of organochlorine insecticides in people of Nigeria. Environm. Physiol. Biochem., 2, 59

Whetstone, R.R. (1964) Chlorocarbons and chlorohydrocarbons: chlorinated derivatives of cyclopentadiene. In: Kirk, R.E. & Othmer, D.F., eds., Encyclopedia of Chemical Technology, 2nd ed., New York, John Wiley & Sons, Vol. 5, p. 240

Wiemeyer, S.N., Mulhern, B.M., Ligas, F.J., Hensel, R.J., Mathisen, J.E., Robards, F.C. & Postupalsky, S. (1972) Residues of organochlorine pesticides, polychlorinated biphenyls and mercury in bald eagle eggs and changes in shell thickness, 1969 and 1970. Pest. Monit. J., 6, 50

Wiersma, G.B., Mitchell, W.G. & Stanford, C.L. (1972a) Pesticide residues in onions and soil - 1969. Pest. Monit. J., 5, 345

Wiersma, G.B., Taï, H. & Sand, P.F. (1972b) Pesticide residue levels in soils, FY 1969 - National Soils Monitoring Program. Pest. Monit. J., 6, 194

Wiersma, G.B., Taï, H. & Sand, P.F. (1972c) Pesticide residues in soil from eight cities - 1969. Pest. Monit. J., 6, 126

Zavon, M.R., Tye, R. & Latorre, L. (1969) Chlorinated hydrocarbon insecticide content of the neonate. Ann. N.Y. Acad. Sci., 160, 196

METHOXYCHLOR

Methoxychlor is the common name approved by the International Standards Organization for 1,1,1-trichloro-2,2-di-(4-methoxyphenyl)ethane. A review on this compound is available (FAO/WHO, 1965).

1. Chemical and Physical Data

1.1 Synonyms and trade names

Chem. Abstr. No.: 72-43-5

2,2-Bis(p-methoxyphenyl)-1,1,1-trichloroethane; dianisyl trichloroethane; 2,2-di-p-anisyl-1,1,1-trichloroethane; dimethoxy-DDT; dimethoxy-DT, di(p-methoxyphenyl)-trichloromethyl methane; DMDT; Marlate; methoxy-DDT; Moxie; 1,1,1-trichloro-2,2-bis(p-methoxyphenyl)ethane; 1,1,1-trichloro-2,2-di(4-methoxyphenyl)ethane

1.2 Chemical formula and molecular weight

$CH_3O-C_6H_4-CH(CCl_3)-C_6H_4-OCH_3$ $C_{16}H_{15}Cl_3O_2$ Mol. wt: 345.7

1.3 Chemical and physical properties of the pure substance

(a) Description: Colourless crystals

(b) Melting-point: 78-78.2°C or 86-88°C (dimorphic)

(c) Solubility: Practically insoluble in water; moderately soluble in ethanol and petroleum oils; readily soluble in most aromatic solvents

(d) Chemical reactivity: Resistant to heat and oxidation and less readily dehydrochlorinated by alcoholic alkalis than DDT

1.4 Technical products and impurities

Technical methoxychlor is a white powder consisting of about 88% of the p,p'-isomer, the remainder being the o,p'-isomer (Martin, 1968).

Methoxychlor is available in the United States as a technical grade product containing 88% of the p,p'-isomer. Also available are wettable powders (50% technical methoxychlor), emulsifiable concentrates, dusts and aerosol sprays; it is frequently formulated with other insecticides such as organophosphates (Berg, 1971).

2. Production, Use, Occurrence and Analysis

2.1 Production and use[1]

Methoxychlor was first synthesized in 1893, although its insecticidal properties were not discovered until 1944 in Germany (Lawless et al., 1972). Commercial production was first reported in the US in 1946 (US Tariff Commission, 1947). Methoxychlor is produced commercially by the condensation of methyl phenyl ether (anisole) with chloral in the presence of sulphuric acid (Merck & Co., 1968).

At least three US companies have reported commercial production of methoxychlor every year since 1968; one source has estimated that 4.5 million kg of methoxychlor were produced in the US in 1971 (Johnson, 1972). Methoxychlor has been used recently in applications where DDT had previously been employed, therefore, the amount produced in recent years may be significantly higher than that produced earlier. Methoxychlor was reportedly made in Israel (US Department of Commerce, 1970) and by one producer in The Netherlands (Economic Documentation Office, 1967) in 1967.

The only known use of methoxychlor is as an insecticide. As of May 31, 1972 it was approved in the US for use on 78 agricultural crops (including several types of seed), with tolerances for residues on the raw agricultural commodities set at 2-100 ppm and with restrictions on the use of treated seeds. Methoxychlor was also approved for use as an insecticide on beef cattle, dairy cattle, goats, sheep and swine and for spray treatment of barns, grain bins, mushroom houses and other agricultural premises (US Environmental Protection Agency, 1972).

---

[1] Data from Chemical Information Services, Stanford Research Institute, USA

Methoxychlor usage in California, a major agricultural state, was reported to have been 50 thousand kg in 1971 (California Department of Agriculture, 1972) and 64 thousand kg in 1972 (over 93% of this was used for the treatment of alfalfa) (California Department of Agriculture, 1973).

The sale of methoxychlor for agricultural purposes has recently been forbidden in Italy.

2.2 Occurrence

(a) Soil and water

Of 1,729 cropland soil samples tested, only one contained detectable levels of methoxychlor (0.28 ppm) (Wiersma et al., 1972). This compound was not detected in water samples at the Jordan River outlet from Lake Utah, probably because of its rapid degradation, but residues of up to 5.2 ppb were found at other sampling stations. Residues found in 2 fish taken from this lake were 56 and 62 ppb (Bradshaw et al., 1972). A median value of <0.01 ppm (drained weight) was found in 6 out of 133 oyster samples (Bugg et al., 1967).

(b) Food

Due to its rapid degradation (Metcalf et al., 1971) and low tissue storage (Weikel, 1957), methoxychlor is found in only trace amounts in food items. In feeding studies in cattle, no residues were found in the body fat of animals fed 25 ppm for 16 weeks (Claborn, 1956), and methoxychlor showed very little tendency to be excreted in the milk, even when dietary concentrations of up to 7000 ppm were given to dairy cows. Feeding of 800 and 7000 ppm in the diet resulted in 0.13 ppm and 2.14 ppm, respectively, in the milk at 16 weeks (Gannon et al., 1959). Duggan (1967) found an average level of 0.001 ppm in dairy products.

The residue on alfalfa 7 days after application of 1 lb/acre was 12.5 ppm, and this decreased to 5.9 ppm after 14 days (Hardee et al., 1963). Miles et al (1964) detected 70 ppm immediately after application of 1 lb/acre; this value decreased to 5.3 ppm after 33 days.

In total diet studies carried out in the US in 1963-1969, only traces of methoxychlor were detected in dairy products (Duggan et al., 1971), while in another study in 1969-1970 the concentration ranged from 0.008-0.059 ppm (Corneliussen, 1972). No methoxychlor was detected in a UK total diet study (Abbott et al., 1969).

The total dietary intake in the US was found to range from 0 (1965) to traces (1966, 1969) to 0.02 µg/kg bw/day (1967, 1968, 1970) (Duggan & Corneliussen, 1972).

The acceptable daily intake for man has been established at 0-0.10 mg/kg bw/day (FAO/WHO, 1965)

2.3 Analysis

A general approach to the analysis of organochlorine pesticides has been given in the preamble (p.16). Weil et al. (1972) describe the determination of methoxychlor in water using accumulation on polyethylene foils.

Other methods used for the detection of methoxychlor in various media can be found in references given in the section on "Occurrence".

3. Biological Data Relevant to the Evaluation of Carcinogenic Risk to Man

3.1 Carcinogenicity and related studies in animals

(a) Oral administration

Rat: In an unpublished study by Nelson & Fitzhugh quoted by Deichmann et al. (1967) 6 groups of 24 Osborne-Mendel rats were fed diets containing 10, 25, 100, 200, 500 and 2000 ppm methoxychlor for 2 years, at which time 52% of the animals were still alive. One rat fed 500 ppm and 5 rats (mainly females) fed 2000 ppm were found to have liver nodules which were diagnosed as non-malignant liver adenomas. All but one liver tumour-bearing animals survived for 2 years. The same study was reported by Lehman (1965) with the comment that "the incidence of tumours was not increased", whereas earlier (Lehmann, 1952) it was reported that a slight increase of hepatic cell adenomas had occurred.

Four groups of 25 male and 25 female rats were fed a diet containing either 0, 25, 200 or 1600 ppm methoxychlor for 2 years. No tumours were found in 13 controls which survived until the end of the experiment. One neurofibroma and 1 lung tumour were found in 13 survivors administered 25 ppm; 1 mammary tumour was found in 10 survivors administered 200 ppm; and 1 mammary tumour, 1 ovarian cystoadenoma, 1 tumour of the abdominal wall, 1 adenocarcinoma of the pancreas and 1 epidermoid carcinoma were found in 16 survivors administered 1600 ppm (Hodge et al., 1952). (The increased number of tumours in animals fed 1600 ppm is considered by the authors to be coincidental; all these tumours, with the exception of the adenocarcinoma of the pancreas, occur commonly in their colony of rats.)

A group of 30 male and 30 female Osborne-Mendel rats was administered a diet containing 80 ppm methoxychlor for 2 years, and a similar group was fed a control diet. Malignant tumours were found in 5 treated and in 9 control rats; benign tumours were present in 8 treated and in 6 control rats. The distribution of tumours by site and type was similar in the two groups (Radomski et al., 1965).

In a 27-month study on 30 male and 30 female Osborne-Mendel rats administered 1000 ppm methoxychlor, 54/60 treated rats were alive at 18 months compared with 48/60 in controls. The incidence and distribution of benign and malignant tumours (mainly mammary and subcutaneous) were similar in treated and control groups (Deichmann et al., 1967).

(b) Skin application

Mouse: Two groups of 50 male and 50 female C3H/Anf mice were painted weekly with doses of either 0.1 or 10 mg methoxychlor in 0.2 ml acetone (the total dose was 0.1-10.4 mg at the low level and 10-980 mg at the high level). The mean survival time ranged from 342 days in females given the low dose to 450 days in the other groups. No skin tumours were observed. Histological observation was limited to 51 treated mice (Hodge et al., 1966).

(c) Subcutaneous and/or intramuscular administration

A group of 50 male and 50 female young adult C3H/Anf mice was given single s.c. injections of 10 mg methoxychlor in 0.02 ml trioctanoin. The mean survival time was 372 days in the males and 419 days in the females. No subcutaneous tumours were observed. Histological observation was confined to 24 mice (Hodge et al., 1966).

3.2 Other relevant biological data

(a) Metabolism and storage in animals

In mice, labelled methoxychlor given orally was eliminated to the extent of 98.3% within 24 hours. 2-(p-Hydroxyphenyl)-2-(p-methoxyphenyl)-1,1,1-trichloroethane and 2,2-bis(p-hydroxyphenyl)-1,1,1-trichloroethane were identified (Metcalf et al., 1970).

Methoxychlor given intravenously to rats is rapidly detoxified by the liver to unidentified hydrophilic metabolites; these are excreted mainly in the bile and a small amount in the urine. Very little reabsorption occurs in the gastrointestinal tract (Weikel, 1957).

Three daily i.p. doses of 50 mg/kg bw methoxychlor increased uterine weight in rats within 18 hours after the last injection and decreased the uptake of oestradiol-17β by the uterus (Welch et al., 1969).

Weanling rats fed 500 ppm methoxychlor in the diet from 4-18 weeks of age stored from 14-36 ppm in their adipose tissue. Equilibrium was reached in 4 weeks, and stored methoxychlor disappeared from the fatty tissue within 2 weeks after cessation of exposure. Rats fed 100 ppm stored from 1-7 ppm. At lower dietary levels, 25 ppm, no methoxychlor was stored. No sex difference in storage was observed in rats (Kunze et al., 1950).

In cows, Cluett et al. (1960) found residues in milk shortly after the cows were sprayed with aqueous suspensions of methoxychlor. A maximum level of 0.1 ppm occurred 1 day after treatment, and detectable levels persisted for one week. Methoxychlor shows little tendency to be stored in body fat or to be excreted in milk.

3.3 Observations in man

No data are available to the Working Group.

4. Comments on Data Reported and Evaluation

4.1 Animal data

Methoxychlor was tested by the oral route only in the rat. Three experiments, including one employing dietary levels of up to 1600 ppm (equivalent to about 80 mg/kg bw/day), provided no evidence of carcinogenicity. Because of inadequate reporting, conclusions cannot be drawn from the results of a fourth experiment in which some liver tumours were observed in rats fed up to 2000 ppm in the diet (equivalent to about 100 mg/kg bw/day). Data from these four experiments do not allow an evaluation of the carcinogenicity of methoxychlor to be made at the present time.

No tumours were reported in limited skin application and subcutaneous injection (single-dose) studies.

4.2 Human data

No epidemiological studies were available to the Working Group.

5. References

Abbott, D.C., Holmes, D.C. & Tatton, J.O'G. (1969) Pesticide residues in the total diet in England and Wales, 1966-1967. II. Organochlorine pesticide residues in the total diet. J. Sci. Fd Agric., 20, 245

Berg, G.L., ed. (1971) Farm Chemicals Handbook, Willoughby, Ohio, Meister p. 228

Bradshaw, J.S., Loveridge, E.L., Rippee, K.P., Peterson, J.L., White, D.A., Barton, R.J. & Fuhriman, D.K. (1972) Seasonal variations in residues of chlorinated hydrocarbon pesticides in the water of the Utah Lake drainage system - 1970 and 1971. Pest. Monit. J., 6, 166

Bugg, J.C., Jr, Higgins, J.E. & Robertson, E.A., Jr (1967) Chlorinated pesticide levels in the eastern oyster (Crassostrea virginica) from selected areas of the South Atlantic and Gulf of Mexico. Pest. Monit. J., 1, iii, 9

California Department of Agriculture (1972) Pesticide Use Report, 1971, Sacramento, pp. 114-115

California Department of Agriculture (1973) Pesticide Use Report, 1972, Sacramento, pp. 127-128

Claborn, H.V. (1956) Insecticide residues in meat and milk. US Department of Agriculture ARS-33-25, Washington DC, US Government Printing Office, p. 30

Cluett, M.L., Lowen, W.K., Pease, H.L. & Woodhouse, C.A. (1960) Determination of methoxychlor and/or metabolites in milk following topical application to dairy cows. J. agric. Fd Chem., 8, 277

Corneliussen, P.E. (1972) Pesticide residues in total diet samples (VI). Pest. Monit. J., 5, 313

Deichmann, W.B., Keplinger, M. Sala, F. & Glass, E. (1967) Synergism among oral carcinogens. IV. The simultaneous feeding of four tumorigens to rats. Toxicol. appl. Pharmacol., 11, 88

Duggan, R.E. (1967) Chlorinated pesticide residues in fluid milk and other dairy products in the United States. Pest. Monit. J., 1, iii, 2

Duggan, R.E. & Corneliussen, P.E. (1972) Dietary intake of pesticide chemicals in the United States (III), June 1968-April 1970. Pest. Monit. J., 5, 331

Duggan, R.E., Lipscomb, G.Q., Cox, E.L., Heatwole, R.E. & Kling, R.C. (1971) Pesticide residue levels in foods in the United States from July 1, 1963 to June 30, 1969. Pest. Monit. J., 5, 73

Economic Documentation Office (1967) *Entoma Europe, 1966-67*, Hilversum, The Netherlands, pp. 212-213

FAO/WHO (1965) Evaluation of the toxicity of pesticide residues in food. FAO/PL:1965/10/1; WHO/Food Add./27.65

Gannon, N., Link, R.P. & Decker, G.C. (1959) Insecticide residues in the milk of dairy cows fed insecticides in their daily ration. *J. agric. Fd Chem.*, 7, 829

Hardee, D.D., Huddleston, E.W. & Gyrisco, G.G. (1963) Initial deposit and disappearance rates of various insecticides as affected by forage crop species. *J. econ. Entomol.*, 56, 98

Hodge, H.C., Maynard, E.A. & Blanchet, H.J., Jr (1952) Chronic oral toxicity tests of methoxychlor (2,2-di-(p-methoxyphenyl)-1,1,1-trichloroethane) in rats and dogs. *J. Pharmacol. exp. Ther.*, 104, 60

Hodge, H.C., Maynard, E.A., Downs, W.L., Ashton, J.K. & Salerno, L.L. (1966) Tests on mice for evaluating carcinogenicity. *Toxicol. appl. Pharmacol.*, 9, 583

Johnson, O. (1972) Pesticides '72. *Chemical Week*, July 26, p. 24

Kunze, F.M., Laug, E.P. & Prickett, C.S. (1950) Storage of methoxychlor in the fat of the rat. *Proc. Soc. exp. Biol. (N.Y.)*, 75, 415

Lawless, E.W., Rumker, R. & Furguson, T.L. (1972) *The Pollution Potential in Pesticide Manufacturing, Pesticide Study Series-5, Technical Studies Report: TS-00-72-04*, US Environmental Protection Agency, Washington DC, US Government Printing Office, p. 6

Lehman, A.J. (1952) Chemicals in food - a report to the association of food and drug officials on current developments. II. Pesticides. V. Pathology. *Quart. Bull. Assoc. Fd & Drugs Officials US*, 16, 126

Lehman, A.J. (1965) *Summaries of pesticide toxicity*, Food & Drug Administration, US Department of Health, Education & Welfare, Washington, DC, US Government Printing Office, pp. 29-31

Martin, H., ed. (1968) *Pesticide Manual*. Basic Information on the Chemicals used as Active Components of Pesticides, 2nd ed., Ombersley, British Crop Protection Council, p. 290

Merck & Co. (1968) *The Merck Index*, 8th ed., Rahway, N.J., p. 677

Metcalf, R.L., Kapoor, I.P., Nystrom, R.F. & Sangha, G.K. (1970) Comparative metabolism of methoxychlor, methiochlor and DDT in mouse, insects and in a model ecosystem. *J. agric. Fd Chem.*, 18, 1145

Metcalf, R.L., Sangha, G.K. & Kapoor, I.P. (1971) Model ecosystem for the evaluation of pesticide biodegradability and ecological magnification. Environm. Sci. Technol., 5, 709

Miles, J.R.W., Sans, W.W., Wressell, H.B. & Manson, G.F. (1964) Growth-dilution as a factor in the decline of pesticide residues of alfalfa-grass forage. Can. J. Plant Sci., 44, 37

Radomski, J.L., Deichmann, W.B., MacDonald, W.E. & Glass, E.M. (1965) Synergism among oral carcinogens. I. Results of the simultaneous feeding of four tumorigens to rats. Toxicol. appl. Pharmacol., 7, 652

US Department of Commerce (1970) Chemicals, June, Washington DC, US Government Printing Office, p. 16

US Environmental Protection Agency (1972) EPA Compendium of Registered Pesticides, Washington DC, US Government Printing Office, pp. III-M-10.1 - III-M-10.9

US Tariff Commission (1947) Synthetic Organic Chemicals, United States Production and Sales, 1946 Second Series, Report No. 159, Washington DC, US Government Printing Office, p. 133

Weikel, J.H., Jr (1957) The metabolism of methoxychlor (1,1,1-trichloro 2,2-bis-(o-methoxyphenyl) ethane). I. The role of the liver and biliary excretion in the rat. Arch. int. Pharmacodyn., 110, 423

Weil, L., Quentin, K.E. & Gitzowa, S. (1972) Zur Analytik der Pestizide im Wasser. IV. Kinetik der Pestizidanreicherung in Polyaethylen. Gas-Wasserfach Wasser-Abwasser, 113, 64

Welch, R.M., Levin, W. & Conney, A.H. (1969) Estrogenic action of DDT and its analogs. Toxicol. appl. Pharmacol., 14, 358

Wiersma, G.B., Taï, H. & Sand, P.F. (1972) Pesticide residue levels in soils, FY 1969 - National Soils Monitoring Program. Pest. Monit. J., 6, 194

MIREX

Mirex is the common name approved by the Entomological Society of America for dodecachloropentacyclo $(3,3,2,0^{2,6},0^{3,9},0^{7,10})$ decane.

1. Chemical and Physical Data

1.1 Synonyms and trade names

Chem. Abstr. No.: 2385-85-5

1,1a,2,2,3,3a,4,5,5,5a,5b,6-Dodecachlorooctahydro-1,3,4-metheno-1H-cyclobuta[c,d]pentalene; dodecachloro-octahydro-1,3,4-metheno-2H-cyclobuta[c,d]pentalene; dodecachloropentacyclo $(3,3,2,0^{2,6},0^{3,9},0^{7,10})$ decane; dodecachloropentacyclodecane; ENT 25719; GC 1283; hexachlorocyclopentadiene dimer; HRS 1276; perchloropentacyclo[5,2,1,0^{2,6},0^{3,9},0^{5,6}]decane

1.2 Chemical formula and molecular weight

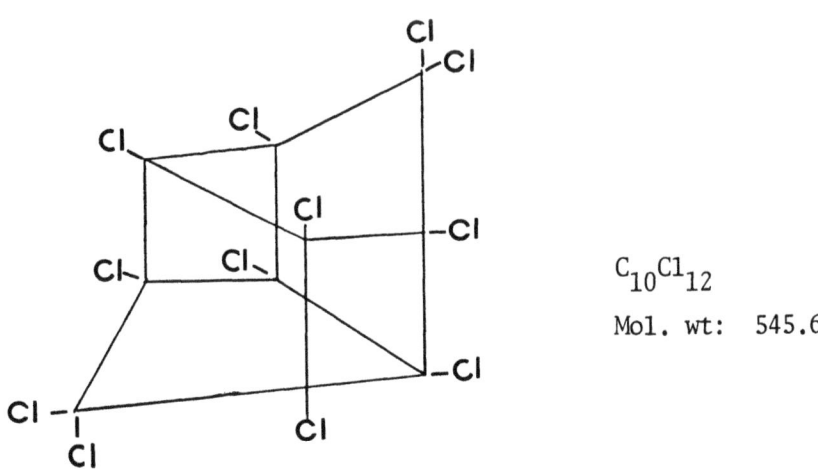

$C_{10}Cl_{12}$

Mol. wt: 545.6

1.3 Chemical and physical properties of the pure substance

(a) <u>Description</u>: Snow-white, odourless crystals

(b) <u>Melting-point</u>: 485°C (decomposes)

(c) _Solubility_: Practically insoluble in water; soluble in benzene, carbon tetrachloride, dioxane, methyl ethyl ketone and xylene

(d) _Chemical reactivity_: Unaffected by sulphuric, nitric or hydrochloric acids

1.4 Technical products and impurities

The only US producer sells the chemical to formulators of insect baits only, thus no information on mirex itself is available. The baits may contain up to 10% mirex but more frequently contain 0.5% or less on a carrier.

2. Production, Use, Occurrence and Analysis

A review article on mirex has been published (Shapley, 1971).

2.1 Production and use[1]

Mirex was first synthesized in the laboratory in the mid-1940's but was not offered for sale in commercial quantities in the US until 1958. It is made by the dimerization of hexachlorocyclopentadiene in the presence of aluminium chloride.

Only one company in the world manufactures mirex, and Johnson (1972) has estimated that less than 454 thousand kg of mirex were produced by this US company in 1971. The amount produced in recent years may be considerably less than that produced in earlier years due to concern about environmental problems.

The only known use for mirex is as an insecticide, and by far the major application to date has been in the control of imported fire ants in the southern US, although it is reportedly also useful against leaf cutters in South America, against harvester termites in South Africa, against Western harvester ants in the US, and has been investigated for use against yellow jackets in the US (Vaughn, 1971). Prior to 1971, it was approved by

---

[1] Data from Chemical Information Services, Stanford Research Institute, USA

the US Department of Agriculture for use on pasture and cropland, and since at least 1968, approximately 11 million acres of land have been treated annually with mirex bait under government-sponsored programmes to control the imported fire ant. The quantity of mirex applied in these programmes was reported to have been 19.4 thousand kg in the fiscal year 1971 (US Department of Agriculture, 1972). However, in March 1971 the US Environmental Protection Agency (EPA) cancelled all federal regulations for its use, pending the outcome of a study of possible residue problems and effects on wildlife. In early 1972, after reviewing the results of the study, the EPA approved the use of mirex in the control of the imported fire ant under tight restrictions on methods and locations of applications; and the quantity applied under government-sponsored programmes in the fiscal year 1972 amounted to 18.8 thousand kg (US Department of Agriculture, 1973). In October 1973 the EPA approved aerial spraying of mirex by the US Department of Agriculture on 12.6 million acres in southeastern US (Anon., 1973).

Tolerances for residues of mirex in food products set by the EPA in 1969 were as follows: 0.1 ppm in fat of meat from cattle, goats, hogs, horses, poultry and sheep; 0.1 ppm in eggs; 0.1 ppm in milk fat; 0.01 ppm in or on all raw agricultural commodities, exclusive of eggs, milk fat and animal fat (US Environmental Protection Agency, 1969).

2.2 Occurrence

Mirex residues have been detected only in animals. The residues present in 10/12 starlings examined ranged from 0.01-1.66 ppm (Oberheu, 1972). Highest concentrations were found in fatty tissue of fish (0-11.2 ppm), of birds (traces-104.4 ppm), of deer (0-0.3 ppm) and of beef (0-0.1 ppm). Concentrations in liver ranged from 0-0.7 ppm for fish and from 0-7.5 ppm for birds; and small quantities have also been detected in brain, heart and eggs of birds. In addition, in 2 out of 3 samples of cow's milk, 0.007 and 0.016 ppm (fat basis) have been found (Baetcke et al., 1972).

In 1970, 1.25 lbs/acre mirex bait were being applied yearly to an estimated 15 million acres of land (US Department of Agriculture, 1971). Within the last few years residues of mirex have been found in various non-target organisms (Butler, 1969; Markin et al., 1969; McKenzie, 1970); Collins et al. (1973) have found mirex residues ranging from 0.008-2.59 ppm in wild catfish from areas which had received a blanket application of mirex bait. In a control experiment in which 1.25 lbs/acre mirex bait were sprayed on a fish pond and its surrounding drainage area, 0.65 ppm mirex had accumulated in uncaged fish after 6 months.

2.3 Analysis

A general approach to the analysis of organochlorine pesticides has been given in the preamble (p. 16).

Uk et al. (1972) describe the use of mass spectrometry for the determination of mirex. A special isolation and clean-up procedure using Florisil columns is described by Porter & Burke (1973) for the determination of low levels of organochlorine pesticide residues, including mirex, in fats and oils by GLC. Details of a collaborative study for the determination of several chlorinated pesticides, including mirex, present in apples and cauliflowers are given by Krause (1973).

3. Biological Data Relevant to the Evaluation of Carcinogenic Risk to Man

3.1 Carcinogenicity and related studies in animals

(a) Oral administration

Mouse: In a study reported as a preliminary note, a group of 18 male and 18 female (C57BL/6 x C3H/Anf)F1 mice and another group with similar numbers of (C57BL/6 x AKR)F1 mice were given single doses of 10 mg/kg bw mirex by stomach tube when the animals were 7 days of age, and this same absolute amount was then given daily until the animals were 28 days of age, when they were tranferred to a diet containing 26 ppm mirex. Treatment continued until 70 weeks, when all mice had died. Hepatomas were observed in both sexes, combined male and female incidences being 14/34 in (C57BL/6 x C3H/Anf) F1 mice and 15/31 in (C57BL/6 x AKR)F1 mice compared with 8/166 and 6/172, respectively, in controls. Females were found to be more susceptible than males. The incidence of other tumours was similar in tested and control animals (Innes et al., 1969).

3.2 Other relevant biological data

(a) Metabolism and storage in animals

When ^{14}C-mirex was administered to rats as single doses of 6 mg/kg bw, more than 50% was excreted unchanged in the faeces within 48 hours, after which time total excretion dropped rapidly. Urinary excretion was very low throughout the experiment; less than 1% was found in the urine after 7 days, and none had been metabolized. Tissue and organs contained about 34% of unchanged mirex 7 days after a single dose. No metabolites were found (Mehendale et al., 1972).

Gibson et al. (1972) reported that rats given single oral doses of 0.2 mg/kg bw ^{14}C-mirex excreted 15.2% in the faeces within 2 days and 2.7% in the subsequent 5 days; none was found in the urine. A concentration of 1 ppm mirex was found in adipose tissue; this level remained unchanged within the next 28 days. Other tissue concentrations were lower and declined within the first 7 days after dosing. A mirex photoproduct, a monohydro derivative, behaved in a similar way to the original compound.

In a reproduction study in rats, mirex was transferred through the placenta and excreted in their milk. Rats fed 25 ppm mirex (2.3 mg/kg bw/day) in their diet for 78 days excreted an arithmetic mean of 11.3 ppm in their milk. A mean of 0.23 ppm mirex was found in foetuses removed on the 19th day of gestation from dams which had been fed 25 ppm mirex (Gaines & Kimbrough, 1970).

4. Comments on Data Reported and Evaluation[1]

4.1 Animal data

Mirex was tested in a preliminary study by the oral route in two strains of mice (the only route and species for which published results were available). It produced an increased incidence of hepatomas in both sexes of both strains used.

---

[1] See also the section "Animal Data in Relation to the Evaluation of Risk to Man" in the introduction to this volume.

4.2 Human data

No epidemiological studies were available to the Working Group.

5. References

Anon. (1973) Mirex aerial spraying is okayed for Southeast. <u>Chemical Marketing Reporter</u>, October 1, p. 4

Baetcke, K.P., Cain, J.D. & Poe, W.E. (1972) Mirex and DDT residues in wildlife and miscellaneous samples in Mississippi, 1970. <u>Pest. Monit. J.</u>, <u>6</u>, 14

Butler, P.A. (1969) Monitoring pesticide pollution. <u>BioScience</u>, <u>19</u>, 889

Collins, H.L., Davis, J.R. & Markin, G.P. (1973) Residues of mirex in channel catfish and other aquatic organisms. <u>Bull. environm. Contam. Toxicol.</u>, <u>10</u>, 73

Gaines, T.B. & Kimbrough, R.D. (1970) Oral toxicity of mirex in adult and suckling rats with notes on the ultrastructure of liver changes. <u>Arch. environm. Hlth</u>, <u>21</u>, 7

Gibson, J.R., Ivie, G.W. & Dorough, H.W. (1972) Fate of mirex and its major photo-decomposition products in rats. <u>J. agric. Fd Chem.</u>, <u>20</u>, 1246

Innes, J.R.M., Ulland, B.M., Valerio, M.G., Petrucelli, L., Fishbein, L., Hart, E.R., Pallotta, A.J., Bates, R.R., Falk, H.L., Gart, J.J., Klein, M., Mitchell, I. & Peters, J. (1969) Bioassay of pesticides and industrial chemicals for tumorigenicity in mice. A preliminary note. <u>J. nat. Cancer Inst.</u>, <u>42</u>, 1101

Johnson, O. (1972) Pesticides '72. <u>Chemical Week</u>, July 26, p. 25

Krause, R.T. (1973) Determination of several chlorinated pesticides by the AOAC multiresidue method with additional quantitation of perthane after dehydrochlorination: collaborative study. <u>J. Ass. off. analyt. Chem.</u>, <u>56</u>, 721

Markin, G.P., Dillier, J.H., Collins, H.L., Wilson, N.L., Spence, J.H., Mauffray, C.J., Murl, M. & Cuevas, M.J. (1969) Quarterly report of research and methods improvement for the imported fire ant. <u>ARS, USDA</u>, <u>69</u>, Washington DC, US Government Printing Office, p. 165

McKenzie, M.D. (1970) <u>Technical Report I.</u> Columbia, SC, South Carolina Wildlife Resources Department, p. 45

Mehendale, H.M., Fishbein, I., Fields, M. & Matthews, H.B. (1972) Fate of mirex-^{14}C in the rat and plants. <u>Bull. environm. Contam. Toxicol.</u>, <u>8</u>, 200

Oberheu, J.C. (1972) The occurrence of mirex in starlings collected in seven southeastern states, 1970. <u>Pest. Monit. J.</u>, <u>6</u>, 41

Porter, M.L. & Burke, J.A. (1973) An isolation and clean-up procedure for low levels of organochlorine pesticide residues in fats and oils. J. Ass. off. analyt. Chem., 56, 733

Shapley, D. (1971) Mirex and the fire ant: decline in fortunes of "perfect" pesticide. Science, 172, 358

Uk, S., Himel, C.M. & Dirks, T.F. (1972) Mass spectral pattern of mirex (dodecachloro-octahydro-1,3,4-metheno-2H-cyclobuta(cd)-pentalene) and of kepone (decachloro-octahydro-1,3,4-metheno-2H-cyclobuta(cd)-pentalen-2-one) and its application in residue analysis. Bull. environm. Contam. Toxicol., 7, 207

US Department of Agriculture (1971) 1970 Progress Report, Plant Protection Division, Washington DC, US Government Printing Office, p. 13

US Department of Agriculture (1972) The Pesticide Review, 1971, Agricultural Stabilization and Conservation Service, Washington DC, US Government Printing Office, p. 12

US Department of Agriculture (1973) The Pesticide Review, 1972, Agricultural Stabilization and Conservation Service, Washington DC, US Government Printing Office, p. 15

US Environmental Protection Agency (1969) EPA Compendium of Registered Pesticides, Vol. III, Insecticides, Acaricides, Molluscicides and Antifouling Compounds, Washington DC, US Government Printing Office, p. III-D-63

Vaughn, W.L. (1971) Mirex: Next on "EEK-ology ban wagon"? Farm Chemicals, April, pp. 46, 48

QUINTOZENE (PENTACHLORONITROBENZENE)

Quintozene is the common name approved by the International Standards Organization for pentachloronitrobenzene (PCNB) (except in Turkey and USSR where the product is known as terrachlor and PKhNB, respectively). A review on this compound is available (FAO/WHO, 1970).

1. Chemical and Physical Data

1.1 Synonyms and trade names

Chem. Abstr. No.: 82-68-8

Botrilex; Brassicol; Folosan; Olpisan; PCNB; terrachlor; Terraclor; Tilcarex; Tritisan

1.2 Chemical formula and molecular weight

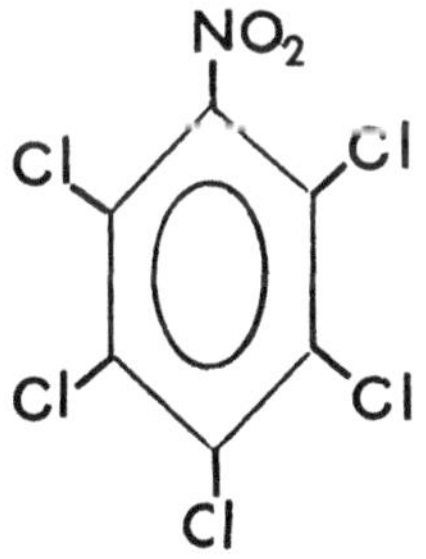

$C_6Cl_5NO_2$ Mol. wt: 295.4

1.3 Chemical and physical properties of the pure substance

(a) Description: Fine, colourless needles or platelets

(b) Melting-point: 146°C

(c) Boiling-point: 328°C (some decomposition)

(d) Solubility: Practically insoluble in water; soluble in ethanol (2% at 25°C); freely soluble in carbon disulphide, benzene and chloroform

(e) Volatility: Vapour pressure is 133×10^{-4} mm Hg at 25°C

(f) Stability: Stable in sunlight

(g) <u>Chemical reactivity</u>: In one study, ultraviolet radiation (2537 Å) resulted primarily in reductive dechlorination; the nitro group was also removed, resulting in the formation of pentachlorobenzene, but corresponding nitroanilines could not be detected (Crosby & Hamadmad, 1971).

1.4 Technical products and impurities

The technical product is 98.5% pure and has a melting-point of 142-145°C. Hexachlorobenzene may be present as an impurity in the quintozene produced by some manufacturers (Borzelleca et al., 1971; Goursaud et al., 1972).

Quintozene is available commercially in the United States, and the technical grade contains 99% minimum active ingredient. The sole US manufacturer also offers a 75% active wettable powder, 10 and 20% active dusts, and various formulations containing 5-ethoxy-3-trichloromethyl-1,2,4-thiadiazole in addition to the quintozene. Other manufacturers supply dusts, wettable powders, emulsifiable concentrates, pastes and formulations containing other pesticides (Frear, 1972).

2. Production, Use, Occurrence and Analysis

2.1 Production and use[1]

The first laboratory synthesis of quintozene was reported in 1868 (Merck & Co., 1968). It was introduced in Germany as a fungicide in the 1930's, but commercial production in the US was not reported until 1962 (US Tariff Commission, 1963). Quintozene is believed to be made commercially by the chlorination of nitrobenzene (Spencer, 1968).

There have been only two companies in the US which have manufactured quintozene and since 1966, only one. Johnson (1972) has estimated that this company produced 1.4 million kg of quintozene in 1971. Imports of quintozene through the principal US customs districts were last reported

---

[1] Data from Chemical Information Services, Stanford Research Institute, USA

for the year 1969 when they amounted to 60 thousand kg (US Tariff Commission, 1970).

One company was reported to be manufacturing quintozene in France in 1973 (Chemical Information Services Ltd., 1973).

The only known use for quintozene is as a fungicide; it is applied both to the soil where crops are grown and as a seed treatment. Although some sources indicate that quintozene can be used for slime prevention in industrial waters and as a herbicide, no indication was found that it is being used for these purposes.

Quintozene is approved in the US for use as a soil fungicide on one fruit (bananas), on a large number of vegetables (e.g., cabbages, potatoes and tomatoes) and on several agricultural field crops (e.g., cotton and soybeans); however, interim tolerances of 0.1 ppm for residues on raw agricultural commodities have been set on most of these crops. Quintozene is also approved in the US for use as a soil fungicide on a large number of ornamental crops (e.g., carnations, grasses, lilies and roses) and as a treatment for use on a wide variety of seeds (e.g., barley, corn, cotton, oats, rice and wheat) (US Environmental Protection Agency, 1973).

Quintozene usage in California, a major agricultural state, was reported to have been 22 thousand kg in 1971 (California Department of Agriculture, 1972) and 25 thousand kg in 1972 (California Department of Agriculture, 1973). Over 70% of the quintozene used in California in 1972 was applied to cotton and about 8% was used for cottonseed treatment.

An indication of possible uses of quintozene can be derived from the FAO/WHO recommended residue limits for quintozene in the following food products: mushrooms, peanuts (whole and kernels), bananas (whole and pulp), lettuces, tomatoes, peppers (bell), broccoli, cabbages, beans (navy and other), potatoes and cottonseed (FAO/WHO, 1973).

2.2 Occurrence

No quintozene could be detected in the milk of dairy cows (St. John et al., 1965), and only traces were found in milk of cows fed 25 mg/day (Goursaud et al., 1972).

In potatoes grown in quintozene-treated soils, the levels of residues increased with the application rate/acre, the highest amount being found in the peel. However, after application of 25 lb/acre, the quintozene concentration did not exceed 0.1 ppm (Easton et al., 1970). Endive leaves and roots were found to contain 0.06-83 ppm of this pesticide (Goursaud et al., 1972).

In the total diet studies, one sample of fruit was found to contain 0.003 ppm quintozene (Duggan et al., 1966; Duggan & Weatherwax, 1967).

2.3 Analysis

Quintozene can be determined by the general methods for organochlorine pesticides described in the preamble (p. 16). A simple and rapid gas chromatographic determination of quintozene in fertilizers is described by Hanks & Engdahl (1972). A GLC method with electron capture detection has been used by Baker & Flaherty (1972) to determine residues in tomatoes, lettuces and bananas. The authors also describe a confirmatory test involving GLC following reduction of the quintozene. For the determination of quintozene residues in food and forage crops, Ackermann et al. (1958) used a spectrophotometric method involving hydrolysis, diazotization and coupling with 1-naphthylamine. An appraisal of three analytical techniques (spectrophotometric, polarographic and microcoulometric gas chromatography) for the determination of quintozene in vegetables has been made by Klein & Gajan (1961).

3. Biological Data Relevant to the Evaluation of Carcinogenic Risk to Man

3.1 Carcinogenicity and related studies in animals

(a) Oral administration

Mouse: In a study reported as a preliminary note, 18 male and 18 female (C57BL/6 x C3H/Anf)F1 mice and similar numbers of (C57BL/6 x AKR)F1 mice were given single doses of 464 mg/kg bw PCNB by stomach tube when the animals were 7 days of age, and this same absolute dose was then given daily until the animals were 28 days of age. The animals were then transferred to a diet containing 1206 ppm PCNB, which was administered up to 78 weeks.

Hepatomas were the only tumours found in excess over the controls; 2/18 male and 4/18 female (C57BL/6 x C3H/Anf)F1 mice developed hepatomas compared with 8/79 and 0/87 controls. Of the (C57BL/6 x AKR)F1 mice, 10/17 males and 1/17 females developed hepatomas compared with 5/90 and 1/82 in controls. The incidence of other tumours was similar in treated and control animals (Innes et al., 1969).

Rat: In a two-year study, groups of 10 male and 10 female rats received diets containing 0, 25, 100, 300, 1000 or 2500 ppm of a commercial preparation containing 20% PCNB. Survival rates were similar in all groups, and at the end of the experiment 41 of the original 120 rats were alive. It is reported that autopsies and histopathological studies were carried out in most animals, but tumour incidences are not given (Finnegan et al., 1958).

(b) Skin application

Mouse: Ten stock albino mice of each sex were painted twice weekly with 0.2 ml of a 0.3% solution of PCNB in acetone for 12 weeks. This was followed by twice-weekly paintings with a 0.5% solution of croton oil in acetone for 20 weeks. In a control group, acetone was given without PCNB. The total number of skin tumours at the end of croton-oil treatment was 12 in 9 surviving controls and 50 in 13 survivors in the PCNB group. One tumour in the PCNB group had progressed to a squamous-cell carcinoma. An infiltrating squamous-cell carcinoma was also observed in 1 control mouse killed 31 weeks from the start of the croton-oil treatment (Searle, 1966).

3.2 Other relevant biological data

(a) Metabolism and storage in animals

After oral administration of 2 g PCNB to rabbits, 62% was found unchanged in the faeces, 12% was excreted as pentachloroaniline and 14% as N-acetyl-S-pentachloro-phenylcysteine (Betts et al., 1955).

After feeding of PCNB (technical grade) over an extended period of time to rats (up to 500 ppm) and beagle dogs (up to 1080 ppm), no PCNB was found in the tissues, but trace amounts of pentachloroaniline and methyl-pentachlorophenylsulphide were detected in various tissues and fat (Borzelleca et al., 1971).

In mice, 4 daily oral doses of PCNB (500 mg/kg bw) led to the appearance of pentachloroaniline and pentachlorophenylsulphide metabolites in fatty tissue of pregnant mice and in foetuses, indicating transplacental passage of these metabolites. PCNB was mainly found in the maternal animals (Courtney, 1973).

3.3 Observations in man

No data were available to the Working Group.

4. Comments on Data Reported and Evaluation[1]

4.1 Animal data

Quintozene (pentachloronitrobenzene) was tested in a preliminary study by the oral route in two strains of mice and produced an increased incidence of hepatomas in males of one strain. A feeding study in rats was considered inadequate. Application of quintozene followed by croton oil to mouse skin gave positive results which could not be interpreted due to a lack of adequate controls.

4.2 Human data

No epidemiological studies were available to the Working Group.

---

[1] See also the section "Animal Data in Relation to the Evaluation of Risk to Man" in the introduction to this volume

5. References

Ackermann, H.J., Baltrush, H.A., Berges, H.H., Brookover, D.O. & Brown, B.B. (1958) Spectrophotometric determination of pentachloronitrobenzene on food and forage crops. J. agric. Fd Chem., 6, 747

Baker, P.B. & Flaherty, B. (1972) Fungicide residues. I. The detection, identification and determination of residues of quintozene in tomatoes, lettuces and bananas by gas chromatography. Analyst, 97, 378

Betts, J.J., James, S.P. & Thorpe, W.V. (1955) The metabolism of pentachloronitrobenzene and 2:3:4:6-tetrachloronitrobenzene and the formation of mercapturic acids in the rabbit. Biochem. J., 61, 611

Borzelleca, J.F., Larson, P.S., Crawford, E.M., Hennigar, G.R., Jr, Kuchar, E.J. & Klein, H.H. (1971) Toxicological and metabolic studies on pentachloronitrobenzene. Toxicol. appl. Pharmacol., 18, 522

California Department of Agriculture (1972) Pesticide Use Report, 1971, Sacramento, p. 138

California Department of Agriculture (1973) Pesticide Use Report, 1972, Sacramento, p. 150

Chemical Information Services, Ltd. (1973) Directory of West European Chemical Producers, Oceanside, NY

Courtney, D. (1973) The effect of pentachloronitrobenzene on fetal kidneys. Toxicol. appl. Pharmacol., 25, 455

Crosby, D.G. & Hamadmad, N. (1971) The photoreduction of pentachloronitrobenzenes. J. agric. Fd Chem., 19, 1171

Duggan, R.E. & Weatherwax, J.R. (1967) Dietary intake of pesticide chemicals. Science, 157, 1006

Duggan, R.E., Barry, H.C. & Johnson, L.Y. (1966) Pesticide residues in total diet samples. Science, 151, 101

Easton, G.D., Maxwell, R.C., Oldenburg, C.R. & Anderson, P.D. (1970) Terrachlor (PCNB) for control of Rhizoctania solani. II. PCNB residues in tubers. Amer. Potat. J., 47, 430

FAO/WHO (1970) 1969 Evaluation of some pesticides in food. FAO/PL/1969/M/17/1; WHO/Food Add./70.38

FAO/WHO (1973) Pesticide residues in food. Report of the 1972 Joint FAO/WHO Meeting. Wld Hlth Org. techn. Rep. Ser., No. 525, p. 40

Finnegan, J.K., Larson, P.S., Smith, R.B., Jr, Haag, H.B. & Hennigar, G.R. (1958) Acute and chronic toxicity studies on pentachloronitrobenzene. Arch. int. Pharmacodyn., 114, 38

Frear, D.E.H., ed. (1972) Pesticide Handbook - Entoma, 24th ed., State College, Pennsylvania, College Science Publishers, p. 178

Goursaud, J., Luquet, F.M., Boudier, J.F. & Casalis, J. (1972) Sur la pollution du lait par les résidus d'hexachlorobenzene (HCB). Ind. Aliment. Agr., 89, 31

Hanks, A.R. & Engdahl, B.S. (1972) Gas chromatographic determination of terrachlor in fertilizers. J. Ass. off. analyt. Chem., 55, 657

Innes, J.R.M., Ulland, B.M., Valerio, M.G., Petrucelli, L., Fishbein, L., Hart, E.R., Pallotta, A.J., Bates, R.R., Falk, H.L., Gart, J.J., Klein, M., Mitchell, I. & Peters, J. (1969) Bioassay of pesticides and industrial chemicals for tumorigenicity in mice. A preliminary note. J. nat. Cancer Inst., 42, 1101

Johnson, O. (1972) Pesticides '72. Chemical Week, July 26, p. 30

Klein, A.K. & Gajan, R.J. (1961) Determination of pentachloronitrobenzene in vegetables. J. Ass. off. analyt. Chem., 44, 712

Merck & Co. (1968) The Merck Index, Rahway, N.J., p. 792

Searle, C.E. (1966) Tumor initiatory activity of some chloromononitrobenzenes and other compounds. Cancer Res., 26, 12

Spencer, E.Y. (1968) Guide to the Chemicals Used in Crop Protection, 5th ed., Ottawa, Canada Department of Agriculture, Research Branch, No. 1093, p. 368

St. John, L.E., Jr, Ammering, J.W., Wagner, D.G. & Lisk, D.J. (1965) Fate of 4,6-dinitro-2-isobutylphenol, 2-chloro-4,6-bis(ethylamino)-S-triazine, and pentachloronitrobenzene in the dairy cow. J. Dairy Sci., 48, 502

US Environmental Protection Agency (1973) Annotated Index of Registered Fungicides and Nematocides, their uses in the United States, Washington DC, US Government Printing Office, pp. I-P-04-00.01 - I-P-04-00.12

US Tariff Commission (1963) Synthetic Organic Chemicals, United States Production and Sales, 1962, TC Publication 114, Washington DC, US Government Printing Office, p. 167

US Tariff Commission (1970) Imports of Benzenoid Chemicals and Products, 1969, TC Publication 328, Washington DC, US Government Printing Office, p. 92

TERPENE POLYCHLORINATES (STROBANE^R)

Strobane^R is a registered name for a mixture of chlorinated terpene isomers.

1. Chemical and Physical Data

1.1 Synonyms and trade names

Chem. Abstr. No.: MX 800 15 01

Chlorinated mixed terpenes; Strobane^R

1.2 Chemical formula and molecular weight

Not applicable (complex mixture)

1.3 Chemical and physical properties of the pure substance

Not applicable (complex mixture)

1.4 Technical products and impurities

The technical product is a straw-coloured liquid with a density of 1.60 and a vapour pressure of 3×10^{-7} mm Hg. It is insoluble in water and soluble in fats and lipid solvents. It is slowly dehydrochlorinated at 100°C and is unstable in the presence of alkalis and organic bases.

Until recently, terpene polychlorinates were available in the United States as a technical product containing a mixture of components resulting from the chlorination of a mixture of camphene and pinene to give a product with 66% chlorine content (Metcalf, 1966). An 80% active concentrate was offered by one formulator (Frear, 1971), and wettable powders and dusts were available. (A related product, chlorinated camphene, Chem. Abstr. Nos. MX 8001352, MX 8022046 and 1319808, is still available in the US under several trade names, e.g., Strobane-T^R and Toxaphene.)

2. Production, Use, Occurrence and Analysis

2.1 Production and use[1]

The date of the first laboratory synthesis of terpene polychlorinates is not known, but commercial production was first reported in 1954 (US Tariff Commission, 1955). Only two US companies have ever produced this product, and no production has been reported since 1969. No estimates of past production were found in the trade literature, but it is believed to have been quite small in the last few years in which it was produced, since it was marketed for many of the same applications as the much more widely used chlorinated camphene.

Terpene polychlorinates were used mainly as an agricultural insecticide, but this product also found some use as a mothproofing agent for woollen clothes. As of May 31, 1969 it was approved as an agricultural insecticide for use on unopened cotton bolls but with restrictions against grazing in treated fields, and the feeding of cotton gin wastes from treated fields to livestock was prohibited. A tolerance of 5.0 ppm residue on cottonseed was in effect. It was also approved for use as a space spray in barns (except in dairy barns and in poultry houses) and in other agricultural premises (US Environmental Protection Agency, 1969).

Terpene polychlorinates usage in California, a major agricultural state, was reported to have been only 81 kg in 1971 (California Department of Agriculture, 1972) and no usage was reported in 1972.

2.2 Occurrence

In milk fat of cows sprayed with terpene polychlorinates, maximum residues of 0.68-0.74 ppm occurred 1 or 2 days after spraying and then decreased to lower values (0.01-0.05 ppm) by 21 days (Claborn et al., 1963).

2.3 Analysis

A general approach to the analysis of organochlorine pesticides has

---

[1] Data from Chemical Information Services, Stanford Research Institute, USA

been given in the preamble (p.16). GLC retention times for various column packing materials were given by Zweig & Sherma (1972) and were compared to those of other organochlorine pesticides. A method based on the titration of organic chlorine in milk samples is described by Claborn et al. (1963).

Residues may be determined by reaction with thiourea in the presence of alkali, the yellow colour being measured at 400 mµ (Hornstein, 1957); the presence of chlordane and heptachlor, however, interferes with this determination.

3. Biological Data Relevant to the Evaluation of Carcinogenic Risk to Man

3.1 Carcinogenicity and related studies in animals

(a) Oral administration

Mouse: In a study reported in a preliminary note, one group of 18 male and 18 female (C57BL/6 x C3H/Anf)Fl mice and another consisting of the same numbers of (C57BL/6 x AKR)Fl mice were given single doses of 4.64 mg/kg bw terpene polychlorinates by stomach tube when the animals were 7 days of age, and this same absolute amount was then given daily until the animals were 28 days old. Subsequently, they were administered a diet containing 11 ppm, and all surviving mice were killed at 80 weeks. Hepatomas were found in 2/15 (C57BL/6 x C3H/Anf)Fl males compared with 8/79 controls, and in 11/18 (C57BL/6 x AKR)Fl males compared with 5/90 controls. No hepatomas were found in females. In addition, 7/33 (5 males and 2 females) (C57BL/6 x C3H/Anf)Fl mice had malignant lymphomas compared with 9/166 in the controls, while no malignant lymphomas were found in treated animals of the other strain (Innes et al., 1969).

3.2 Other relevant biological data

No data were available to the Working Group.

3.3 Observations in man

No data were available to the Working Group.

4. Comments on Data Reported and Evaluation[1]

4.1 Animal data

Terpene polychlorinates (Strobane^R) were tested in a preliminary study by the oral route in two strains of mice and produced an increased incidence of hepatomas in males of one strain. The suggestion that the product also increased the incidence of malignant lymphomas in this species awaits confirmation.

No adequate data were available for other species or other routes of administration.

4.2 Human data

No epidemiological studies were available to the Working Group.

---

[1] See also the section "Animal Data in Relation to the Evaluation of Risk to Man" in the introduction to this volume

5. References

California Department of Agriculture (1972) Pesticide Use Report, 1971, Sacramento, p. 178

Claborn, H.V., Mann, H.D., Ivey, M.C., Radeleff, R.D. & Woodard, G.T. (1963) Excretion of toxaphene and strobane in milk of dairy cows. J. agric. Fd Chem., 11, 286

Frear, D.E.H., ed. (1971) Pesticide Handbook - Entoma, 23rd ed., State College, Pennsylvania, College Science Publishers, p. 192

Hornstein, I. (1957) Colorimetric determination of toxaphene. J. agric. Fd Chem., 5, 446

Innes, J.R.M., Ulland, B.M., Valerio, M.G., Petrucelli, L., Fishbein, L., Hart, E.R., Pallotta, A.J., Bates, R.R., Falk, H.L., Gart, J.J., Klein, M., Mitchell, I. & Peters, J. (1969) Bioassay of pesticides and industrial chemicals for tumorigenicity in mice. A preliminary note. J. nat. Cancer Inst., 42, 1101

Metcalf, R.L. (1966) Insecticides. In: Kirk, R.E. & Othmer, D.F., eds., Encyclopedia of Chemical Technology, 2nd ed., New York, John Wiley & Sons, Vol. 11, p. 695

US Environmental Protection Agency (1969) EPA Compendium of Registered Pesticides, Washington DC, US Government Printing Office, p. III-T-2

US Tariff Commission (1955) Synthetic Organic Chemicals, United States Production and Sales, 1954 Series, Report No. 196, Washington DC, US Government Printing Office, p. 136

Zweig, G. & Sherma, J. (1972) Gas chromatographic analysis. In: Zweig, G., ed., Analytical Methods for Pesticides and Plant Growth Regulators, Vol. VI, New York, London, Academic Press

APPENDIX

ORGANOCHLORINE PESTICIDE RESIDUES IN HUMAN FAT IN
VARIOUS COUNTRIES (MEAN RESIDUES IN PPM)

COUNTRY	PERIOD	LINDANE	TOTAL BHC	DDT
Argentina	1967	0.03^1	2.43^1	-
Austria	1971	0.04^2	-	1.2^2
W. Australia	1965-66 1968	0.25^3 $0-0.33^4$	0.68^3 $0-2.6^4$	- -
Brazil	1969-70	-	0.25^5 (β-BHC)	1.65^5
Bulgaria	-	-	-	-
Canada	1958-60 1970 1967-68	- - -	- - 1.07^9 (α-BHC)	- - 1.56^9 (p,p'-DDT)
Czechoslovakia	- 1963-64	- -	9.78^{10} -	- 5.5^{11}
Denmark	1965	-	-	0.6^{12}
France	1961 1969 1970	- - $0.04-0.05^{15}$	- 0.15^{14} $0.05-0.07^{15}$ (α-BHC)	1.7^{13} 1.9^{14} $0.65-0.75^{15}$ (p,p'-DDT)

p,p'-DDE	TOTAL DDT	DIELDRIN	HEPTACHLOR EPOXIDE
-	13.17^1	0.38^1	0.19^1
4.6^2	5.8^2	0.1^2	-
-	9.3^3	0.67^3	0.02^3
-	-	-	$0-0.5^4$
5.19^5	7.88^5	0.13^5	0.04^5
-	10.06^6	-	-
-	4.9^7	-	-
-	9.22^8	0.22^8	-
4.16^9	-	0.12^9	0.14^9
-	20.34^{10}	-	-
3.7^{11}	-	-	-
2.5^{12}	3.3^{12}	0.2^{12}	-
3.2^{13}	5.2^{13}	-	-
-	5.2^{14}	-	0.15^{14}
$1.87-1.97^{15}$	$3.02-3.37^{15}$	$0.36-0.43^{15}$	$0.28-0.36^{15}$

APPENDIX (cont'd)

COUNTRY	PERIOD	LINDANE	TOTAL BHC	DDT
Federal Republic of Germany	1958-59 1967 -	- 0.03^{17} -	- 0.56^{17} (β&γ-BHC) 0.45^{18} (β-BHC)	1^{16} 1.16^{17} 1.1^{18}
German Democratic Republic	1966	0.01-0.15^{19}	-	3.7^{19}
Hungary	1969	0.99^{20}	2.3^{20} (β&γ-BHC)	5.57^{20}
Israel	1963-64 1965-66	- -	- -	8.5^{21} 8.2^{22}
India (Delhi)	1964 1964	- -	0.86^{23} (α&β-BHC) 1.7^{23} (α&β-BHC)	4.7^{23} 14.2^{23}
Italy	1966 - 1966-69	0.08^{24} 0.01^{25} -	- 2.24^{25} (β-BHC) -	- 2.58^{25} (p,p'-DDT) 1.48^{26}
Japan	- - 1971	0.12^{27} - 0.025^{29}	1.54^{27} 4.26^{28} 2.42^{29}	0.62^{27} - -

p,p'-DDE	TOTAL DDT	DIELDRIN	HEPTACHLOR EPOXIDE
1.17[16]	2.18[16]	-	-
2.4[17]	4.1[17]	0.18[17]	0.05[17]
2.2[18]	3.3[18]	-	-
8.5[19]	13.1[19]	-	-
6.74[20]	-	-	-
10.7[21] (as DDT)	19.2[21]	-	-
9.9[22] (as DDT)	18.1[22]	-	-
6.4[23]	13.7[23]	0.06[23]	-
11.6[23]	30.2[23]	0.03[23]	-
-	15.48[24]	0.68[24]	0.23[24]
7.43[25]	-	0.84[25]	0.46[25]
6.11[26]	9.26[26]	0.07[26]	-
1.78[27]	2.47[27]	0.13[27]	0.02[27]
-	8.11[28]	-	-
-	4.22[29]	0.163[29]	-

APPENDIX (cont'd)

COUNTRY	PERIOD	LINDANE	TOTAL BHC	DDT
Kenya	1969-70	-	0.26^{30} (β-BHC)	-
Netherlands	1967-68	0.10^{31}	-	0.29^{31} (p,p'-DDT)
New Zealand	1965-69 1965 1969 1963-64	0.02^{32} - - 0.02^{33}	- - - 0.5^{33}	- 2.42^{32} 1.04^{32} -
Nigeria	1969	$0.03-0.06^{34}$	$0.16-0.30^{34}$	-
Norway	1970	-	-	-
Poland	- -	- -	0.13^{36} -	4.08^{36} 4.7^{37}
South Africa	1969	0.75^{38}	2.41^{38}	0.9^{38}
UK	1963-64 1965-67 1969-71	- - -	0.42^{39} 0.31^{40} 0.29^{41}	1.1^{39} 0.78^{40} 0.52^{41}

p,p'-DDE	TOTAL DDT	DIELDRIN	HEPTACHLOR EPOXIDE
-	4.5^{30}	0.08^{30}	0.07^{30}
1.26^{31}	1.75^{31}	0.17^{31}	0.0085^{31}
- 5.42^{32} 3.92^{32} -	- - - -	- 0.41^{32} 0.27^{32} -	- - - -
$1.4-2.5^{34}$	6.5^{34}	$0.02-0.18^{34}$	$0.004-0.02^{34}$
-	5.0^{35} (4.67-5.34)	-	-
7.28^{36} 7.45	- -	- -	- -
4.57^{38}	6.38^{38}	0.039^{38}	0.01^{38}
2.0^{39} 2.0^{40} 1.8^{41}	3.3^{39} 3^{40} 2.5^{41}	0.26^{39} 0.21^{40} 0.16^{41}	- 0.04^{40} 0.03^{41}

APPENDIX (cont'd)

COUNTRY	PERIOD	LINDANE	TOTAL BHC	DDT
USA	1966 1962-66 1968	- - -	- 0.48^{43} -	2.81^{42} 2.6^{43} 1.54^{44}

p,p'-DDE	TOTAL DDT	DIELDRIN	HEPTACHLOR EPOXIDE
6.67[42]	10.56[42]	0.22[42]	-
7[43]	-	0.14[43]	0.16[43]
4.58[44]	-	0.14[44]	-

References

1. Wassermann, M., Francone, M.P., Wassermann, D., Mariani, F. & Groner, J. (1969) Contenido en pesticidas órganoclorados en el tejido adiposo de la población general de la República Argentina. La Semana Medica, 134, 7 April, 459

2. Pesendorfer, H., Eichler, I. & Glofke, E. (1973) Orientierende Untersuchungen über Rückstände an DDT, anderen Organochlorpestiziden und PCBs in Humanfettproben. Wien. Klin. Wschr., 85, 218

3. Wassermann, M., Curnow, D.H., Forte, P.N. & Groner, Y. (1968) Storage of organochlorine pesticides in the body fat of people in West Australia. Industr. Med. Surg., 37, 295

4. Brady, M.N. & Siyali, D.S. (1972) Hexachlorobenzene in human body fat. Med. J. Austr., i, 158

5. Wassermann, M., Nogueira, D.P., Tomatis, L., Athie, E., Wassermann, D., Djavaherian, D. & Guttel, C. (1972) Storage of organochlorine pesticides in people of Sao Paulo, Brazil. Industr. Med. Surg., 41, 22

6. Kaloyanova, F., Mikhailova, Zl., Gheorghiev, G.K., Benchev, Iv., Rizov, N. & Velichkova, V. (1972) Organochlorine insecticides in the blood and fat of the Bulgarian people. In: Fifth International Congress on Rural Medicine, Varna, 1972

7. Read, S.T. & McKinley, W.P. (1961) DDT and DDE content of human fat. Arch. environm. Hlth, 3, 209

8. Mastromatteo, E. (1971) Pesticides and man's health. The picture in Ontario. In: Conference of Epidemiology and Toxicology of Pesticides, Amsterdam, 1971

9. Kadis, V.W., Breitkreitz, W.E. & Jonasson, O.J. (1970) Insecticide levels in human tissues of Alberta residents. Canad. J. Publ. Hlth, 61, 413

10. Rosival, L., Szokolay, A., Gorner, F., Madaric, A. & Uhnak, J. (1970) Exposure to pesticides and protection of health of the population. In: Kuroiwa, H., ed., Proceedings of the Fourth International Congress on Rural Medicine, Whither Rural Medicine, Usada, 1969, Tokyo, Japanese Association for Rural Medicine, pp. 40-42

11. Halack, H., Hakl, J. & Vymetal, F. (1965) Effect of massive doses of DDT on human adipose tissues. Cs. Hyg., 10, 188

12. Weihe, M. (1966) Klorerede insekticider i fedtvaev fra mennesker (Chlorinated insecticides in the body fat of people of Denmark). Ugeskr. Laeg., 128, 881

13. Hayes, W.S., Jr, Dale, W.E. & LeBreton, R. (1963) Storage of pesticides in French people. Nature (Lond.), 199, 1189

14. Fournier, E. (1971) Impregnation par pesticides des êtres humains. Cah. Nutr. Diet., 6, 31

15. Fournier, E., Treich, I., Campagne, L. & Capelle, N. (1972) Pesticides organo-chlorés dans le tissu adipeux d'êtres humains en France. Europ. J. Toxicol., 5, 11

16. Maier-Bode, H. (1960) DDT in Körperfett des Menschen. Med. exp. (Basel), 1, 146

17. Wünscher, K. & Acker, L. (1969) Über das Vorkommen von chlorierten Insektiziden im Fettgewebe des Menschen. Med. Ernährung, 10, 5

18. Acker, L. & Schulte, E. (1970) Über das Vorkommen von chlorierten Biphenylen und Hexachlorbenzol neben chlorierten Insektiziden in Humanmilch und menschlichem Fettgewebe. Naturwissenschaften, 57, 497

19. Engst, R., Knoll, R. & Nickel, B. (1967) Über die Anreicherung von chlorierten Kohlenwasserstoffen, insbesondere von DDT und seinem Metaboliten DDE, im menschlichen Fett. Pharmazie, 22, 654

20. Berend, E., Kecskeméti, I. & Koppa, G. (1970) Chlorinated hydrocarbons in human tissues in Veszprém country. Egészségtudomány, 14, 388

21. Wassermann, M., Gon, M., Wassermann, D. & Zellermayer, L. (1965) DDT and DDE in the body fat of people in Israel. Arch. environm. Hlth, 11, 375

22. Wassermann, M., Wassermann, D., Zellermayer, L. & Gon, M. (1967) Storage of DDT in the people of Israel. Pest. Monit. J., 1, ii, 15

23. Dale, W.E., Copeland, M.F. & Hayes, W.J., Jr (1965) Chlorinated insecticides in the body fat of people in India. Bull. Wld Hlth Org., 33, 471

24. Del Vecchio, V. & Leoni, V. (1967) La ricerca ed il dosaggio degli insetticidi clorurati in materiale biologico. II. Gli insetticidi clorurati nei tessuti adiposi di alcuni gruppi della popolazione italiana. Nuovi Ann. Ig. Microbiol., 18, 107

25. Paccagnella, B., Prati, L. & Cavazzini, G. (1967) Insetticidi cloroderivati organici nel tessuto adiposo di persone residenti nella provincia di Ferrara. Nuovi Ann. Ig. Microbiol., 18, 17

26. Prati, L., Pavanello, R. & Ghezzo, F. (1972) Storage of chlorinated pesticides in human organs and tissues in Ferrara Province, Italy. Bull. Wld Hlth Org., 46, 363

27. Curley, A., Burse, V.W., Jennings, R.W., Villanueva, E.C., Tomatis, L. & Akazaki, K. (1973) Chlorinated hydrocarbon pesticides and related compounds in adipose tissue from people of Japan. Nature (Lond.), 242, 338

28. Kasai, A. (1972) Organochlorine insecticide residues in human bodies versus their residues in food. In: Fifth International Congress on Rural Medicine, Varna, 1972

29. Tatsumi, M., Sugaya, T., Sasaki, S., Suzuki, Y. & Sato, T. (1972) Pesticide residues in human milk and fat tissues. In: Fifth International Congress on Rural Medicine, Varna, 1972

30. Wassermann, M., Rogoff, M.G., Tomatis, L., Day, N.E., Wassermann, D., Djavaherian, M. & Guttel, C. (1972) Storage of organochlorine insecticides in the adipose tissue of people in Kenya. Ann. Soc. belge Méd. trop., 52, 509

31. De Vlieger, M., Robinson, J., Baldwin, M.K., Crabtree, A.N. & van Dijk, M.C. (1968) The organochlorine insecticide content of human tissues. Arch. environm. Hlth, 17, 759

32. Copplestone, J.F., Hunnego, J.N. & Harrison, D.L. (1973) Organochlorine insecticide levels in adult New Zealanders. A five-year study. N.Z. J. Sci., 16, 27

33. Dacre, J.C. (1969) Residual metabolites of hexachlorocyclohexane in human adipose tissues. Proc. Univ. Otago Med. School, 47, 74

34. Wassermann, M., Sofoluwe, G.O., Tomatis, L., Day, N.E., Wassermann, D. & Lazarovici, S. (1971) Storage of organochlorine pesticides in people of Nigeria. Environm. Physiol. Biochem., 2, 59

35. Bjerk, J.E. (1972) DDT and polychlorinated biphenyl residues in human material in Norway. Tidsskz. Norske Laegeforen., 92, 15

36. Juszkiewicz, T. & Stec, J. (1971) Residues of chlorinated hydrocarbon insecticides in adipose tissue in peasants from the province of Lublin. Polski Tygodnik Lekarski, 26, 462

37. Trojanowska, M., Stankiewicz, Z., Szucki, B., Pomorska, K. & Majewska, B. (1972) DDT and DDE content of human tissues. Forens. Sci., 1, 239

38. Wassermann, M., Wassermann, D., Lazarovici, S., Coetzee, A.M. & Tomatis, L. (1970) Present state of the storage of the organochlorine insecticides in the general population of South Africa. S.A. med. J., 44, 646

39. Egan, H., Goulding, R., Roburn, G. & Tatton, J.O'G. (1965) Organochlorine pesticide residues in human fat and human milk. Brit. med. J., ii, 66

40. Abbott, D.C., Goulding, R. & Tatton, J.O'G. (1968) Organochlorine pesticide residues in human fat in Great Britain. Brit. med. J., iii, 146

41. Abbott, D.C., Collins, G.B. & Goulding, R. (1972) Organochlorine pesticide residues in human fat in the United Kingdom, 1969-71. Brit. med. J., ii, 553

42. Fiserova-Bergerova, V., Radomski, J.L., Davies, J.E. & Davis, J.H. (1967) Levels of chlorinated hydrocarbon pesticides in human tissues. Industr. Med. Surg., 36, 65

43. Hoffman, W.S., Adler, H., Fishbein, W.I. & Bauer, F.C. (1967) Relation of pesticide concentrations in fat to pathological changes in tissues. Arch. environm. Hlth, 15, 758

44. Morgan, D.P. & Roan, C.C. (1970) Chlorinated hydrocarbon pesticide residues in human tissues. Arch. environm. Hlth, 20, 452

CUMULATIVE INDEX TO IARC MONOGRAPHS ON THE EVALUATION
OF CARCINOGENIC RISK OF CHEMICALS TO MAN

Numbers underlined indicate volume and numbers in italics indicate page.

Aflatoxin B1	1,*145*
Aflatoxin B2	1,*145*
Aflatoxin G1	1,*145*
Aflatoxin G2	1,*145*
Aldrin	5,*25*
4-Aminobiphenyl	1,*74*
Aniline	4,*27*
Aramite^R	5,*39*
Arsenic	2,*48*
Arsenic pentoxide	2,*48*
Arsenic trioxide	2,*48*
Asbestos	2,*17*
Auramine	1,*69*
Benz(c)acridine	3,*241*
Benz(a)anthracene	3,*45*
Benzidine	1,*80*
Benzo(b)fluoranthene	3,*69*
Benzo(j)fluoranthene	3,*82*
Benzo(a)pyrene	3,*91*
Benzo(e)pyrene	3,*137*
Beryl	1,*18*
Beryllium	1,*17*
Beryllium oxide	1,*17*
Beryllium sulphate	1,*18*
BHC (technical grades)	5,*47*
N,N'-Bis(2-chloroethyl)-2-naphthylamine	4,*119*
Bis(chloromethyl)ether	4,*231*
1,4-Butanediol dimethanesulphonate	4,*247*

Cadmium	2,74
Cadmium carbonate	2,74
Cadmium chloride	2,74
Cadmium oxide	2,74
Cadmium sulphate	2,74
Cadmium sulphide	2,74
Calcium arsenate	2,48
Calcium arsenite	2,48
Calcium chromate	2,100
Carbon tetrachloride	1,53
Chlorobenzilate	5,75
Chloroform	1,61
Chloromethyl methyl ether	4,239
Chromic oxide	2,100
Chromium	2,100
Chromium dioxide	2,101
Chromium trioxide	2,101
Chrysene	3,159
Cycasin	1,157
DDD	5,83
DDE	5,83
DDT	5,83
o-Dianisidine	4,41
Dibenz(a,h)acridine	3,247
Dibenz(a,j)acridine	3,254
Dibenz(a,h)anthracene	3,178
7H-Dibenzo(c,g)carbazole	3,260
Dibenzo(h,rst)pentaphene	3,197
Dibenzo(a,e)pyrene	3,201
Dibenzo(a,h)pyrene	3,207
Dibenzo(a,i)pyrene	3,215
Dibenzo(a,l)pyrene	3,224
3,3'-Dichlorobenzidine	4,49
Dieldrin	5,125

1,2-Diethylhydrazine	<u>4</u>,153
Diethyl sulphate	<u>4</u>,277
Dihydrosafrole	<u>1</u>,170
3,3'-Dimethoxybenzidine	<u>4</u>,41
3,3'-Dimethylbenzidine	<u>1</u>,87
1,1-Dimethylhydrazine	<u>4</u>,137
1,2-Dimethylhydrazine	<u>4</u>,145
Dimethyl sulphate	<u>4</u>,271
Endrin	<u>5</u>,157
Haematite	<u>1</u>,29
Heptachlor	<u>5</u>,173
Hydrazine	<u>4</u>,127
Indeno(1,2,3-cd)pyrene	<u>3</u>,229
Iron-dextran complex	<u>2</u>,161
Iron-dextrin complex	<u>2</u>,161
Iron oxide	<u>1</u>,29
Iron-sorbitol-citric acid complex	<u>2</u>,161
Isonicotinic acid hydrazide	<u>4</u>,159
Isosafrole	<u>1</u>,169
Lead acetate	<u>1</u>,40
Lead arsenate	<u>1</u>,41
Lead carbonate	<u>1</u>,41
Lead chromate	<u>2</u>,101
Lead phosphate	<u>1</u>,42
Lead subacetate	<u>1</u>,40
Lindane	<u>5</u>,47
Magenta	<u>4</u>,57
Maleic hydrazide	<u>4</u>,173
Methoxychlor	<u>5</u>,193
Methylazoxymethanol acetate	<u>1</u>,164
N-Methyl-N,4-dinitrosoaniline	<u>1</u>,141
4,4'-Methylene bis (2-chloroaniline)	<u>4</u>,65
4,4'-Methylene bis (2-methylaniline)	<u>4</u>,73
4,4'-Methylenedianiline	<u>4</u>,79

N-Methyl-N'-nitro-N-nitrosoguanidine	4,*183*
Mirex	5,*203*
1-Naphthylamine	4,*87*
2-Naphthylamine	4,*97*
Nickel	2,*126*
Nickel acetate	2,*126*
Nickel carbonate	2,*126*
Nickel carbonyl	2,*126*
Nickelocene	2,*126*
Nickel oxide	2,*126*
Nickel subsulphide	2,*126*
Nickel sulphate	2,*127*
4-Nitrobiphenyl	4,*113*
N-[4-(5-Nitro-2-furyl)-2-thiazolyl]acetamide	1,*181*
N-Nitroso-di-n-butylamine	4,*197*
N-Nitrosodiethylamine	1,*107*
N-Nitrosodimethylamine	1,*95*
Nitrosoethylurea	1,*135*
Nitrosomethylurea	1,*125*
N-Nitroso-N-methylurethane	4,*211*
Pentachloronitrobenzene	5,*211*
Potassium arsenate	2,*48*
Potassium arsenite	2,*49*
Potassium dichromate	2,*101*
1,3-Propane sultone	4,*253*
β-Propiolactone	4,*259*
Quintozene	5,*211*
Saccharated iron oxide	2,*161*
Safrole	1,*169*
Sodium arsenate	2,*49*
Sodium arsenite	2,*49*
Sodium dichromate	2,*102*
Sterigmatocystin	1,*175*

Streptozotocin	<u>4</u>,*221*
Strobane^R	<u>5</u>,*219*
TDE	<u>5</u>,*83*
Terpene polychlorinates	<u>5</u>,*219*
Tetraethyllead	<u>2</u>,*150*
Tetramethyllead	<u>2</u>,*150*
o-Tolidine	<u>1</u>,*87*

www.ingramcontent.com/pod-product-compliance
Ingram Content Group UK Ltd.
Pitfield, Milton Keynes, MK11 3LW, UK
UKHW051259180426
11947UKWH00020B/1797